INTEF

FASTING 16-8

LIFESTYLE

GUIDE

Complete Weight Loss And Healthy

Living Guide+ Starter Meal

by

Josh Smith

TABLE OF CONTENTS

INTRODUCTION

In the world of health, nutrition, and weight loss, intermittent fasting has been getting quite a bit of press in the last few years. Intermittent Fasting is used to denote a specific eating pattern that rotates between periods of eating and fasting. The concept of intermittent fasting is not a regular diet plan. Instead, it is more of an eating pattern and I'm going to talk about here.

This book is to help you decide which fasting protocol is best for you and to help you understand how intermittent fasting works. It will explore the common myths, struggles and benefits, as well as provide guidelines for practices that can aid you in fasting and help you to be successful if and when you choose to endeavor on the program of intermittent fasting.

The different types of fasting and why Intermittent fasting is the right choice for you will be discussed. The information provided here is centered on how Intermittent fasting works.

Intermittent fasting is not a new concept, but it has recently become more widely used, and I wanted to put this book together to help you along this newly chosen path.

CHAPTER 1:

What Is Intermittent Fasting?

Intermittent fasting means not eating for a designated period or a set number of hours and then eating during a time restricted feeding period. Intermittent fasting is proving to be highly beneficial to people's health. There are countless benefits to participating in the lifestyle. Unlike the traditional diet, it focuses more on when you eat as opposed to what you eat. There are many ways to use fasting to your benefit and various techniques you can implement.

There is evidence of benefits on many body systems, including slowing down aging, improving cardiac health, focus, weight loss, along with multiple other benefits. While the vast majority of people are interested in intermittent fasting to aid in weight loss, this guide goes over the other perks of the lifestyle, as well. Unfortunately, there is some negative stigma surrounding intermittent fasting.

Intermittent fasting can best be described as utilizing alternating intervals of fasting and feeding. The idea behind it is that you eat whatever you want, whenever you want during the feeding stage and avoid taking anything with caloric value when in the fasting stage. We will discuss exactly how this affects your body and what the best practices are.

There are several different methods of intermittent fasting that you may choose from. Most people tend to start with lower alternating periods and slowly increase them. Intermittent fasting is fairly easy, and many people report having more energy and feeling better overall during their fasting periods.

Of course, many of us ignore our body's signals in an attempt to lose weight, only to end up binge eating then follow that with under eating, starvation, and binging again. A cycle like this can wreak havoc with your hormones, halt ovulation, affect your menstruation, and even shrink your ovaries. On top of that, it can exacerbate eating disorders, such as; bulimia, anorexia, and binge eating.

CHAPTER 2:

The History Of Intermittent Fasting

Fasting has been around nearly as long as humanity itself. Many ancient written sources have shown that "starvation" has been used in various cultures, countries, and ancient civilizations to help the body recover and restore itself. It seems they were taking advantage of the benefits long before modern times. Ancient India, Greece, and Rome, in particular, used intermittent fasting, not only to strengthen the body but also to help prevent diseases. Back in ancient times, when hunting and berry gathering was one of the primary sources of food, there were periods where nothing could be found, so natural fasting took place. Involuntary fasting caused the hunters and gatherers to be inadvertently and greatly strengthened by the gaps in sustenance. The ancient Greeks mainly believed medical treatments and cures could be found and were observed in nature. When humans, dogs, cats, and most animals are sick, they do not want to eat. This is considered the internal physician in some cultures; it is believed that the body is instinctually fasting to help to heal itself. The ancient Greeks also believed fasting helped to improve mental and cognitive function. This makes sense if you think about when you eat a big meal and feel sleepy and tired or have "food coma" as many like to call it, versus when you are fasting and your brain hyper-focuses on the task at hand. The practices of controlled starvation are essential in many of the world's religions, proving self-control, and penitence. Many religions practice fasting for periods, such as Ramadan in the Islamic culture where they do not eat from sunup to sundown. Christianity recognizes the forty days of lent, which represents the time that Jesus Christ fasted. Fasting is recognized in Islamic religions, Buddhism, Christianity, and countless others.

During Ramadan for example, Muslims fast during the daylight hours, finally eating only once the sun has set. While it sounds terrible at first, many report they feel better after a few days of the practice. This is because they adjust to the schedule and their bodies learn to adapt to no food for some time. This is exactly what intermittent fasting is about.

Science is now beginning to prove what was already known in ancient times. The multiple and seemingly endless benefits keep climbing.

CHAPTER 3:

The Science Behind Intermittent Fasting

For several decades, scientists have been arguing that intermittent fasting makes evolutionary sense. When people went to the forest and successfully hunted an animal, it meant that they had two or three days of feasting on a diet that was rich in calories(meat). However, when the feast was over, they fed themselves with low-calorie roots, berries, and grains. In turn, that led over many years to metabolic or biochemical adaptation. This was through a natural selection process that maximized the survival capacity in those uncertain food supply circumstances.

Remember that our protein, fat and carbohydrate metabolic pathways are similar to the metabolic pathways of bonobos, gorillas, and chimps -our close relatives - who did not adapt to intermittent variations of calories supply. There are essential adaptations that impact the results of intermittent fasting. Intermittent fasting lowers your metabolic rate precisely. This is because your metabolism is structured in such a way that it can conserve energy that is related to the uneven supply of calories in the body.

The challenge is that it works in the opposite direction of people opting for intermittent fasting to burn a higher number of calories.

At face value, it is a challenge to invoke the aspect of hunter-gatherer's paradigm. For more than ten thousand years when man invented agriculture, the supply of calories has been plenty and predictable. People have not lost their metabolic adaptation of energy conservation, but they have gotten progressively plumper and recently even obese.

What does this mean, physiologically? It means that human's metabolic setpoint is higher as compared to the ancient times of hunting and gathering and that hormones are geared to maintain physiological stability that will resist any change in the metabolic set point which we are all aware of.

When it comes to the metabolism theory of hunters and gatherers a more complex side of their diet to consider is the benefits to their overall gut health. Note that obesity can cause a radical change in the gut flora. Moreover, the new gut flora may promote further obesity. Maybe hunters and gatherers did not have this challenge.

Scientific Evidence

The study of intermittent fasting was first employed by Panda and his colleagues from the Salk Institute. Most of the human body functions are controlled by a master pacemaker that is situated in the brain structure known as the suprachiasmatic nucleus. The pacemaker gets a neutral signal from your eyes, and therefore, it is primarily controlled by light and dark periods. In a similar arrangement to your federal system, every organ in your body has its sub-pacemaker designed to serve the particular requirement of that specific organ.

In his research, when he withdrew food from mice for 24 hours period, he found that about 90% of the genes in the liver that were under the circadian regulation of the clock stopped functioning. It is not surprising because we would expect the significant metabolism organs to be controlled by the supply of food.

On the other hand, we can let the mice consume a high-fat diet for 24 hours in a day, and you will find that the same genes become activated around the clock. The result of his study was that the mice became obese, and this explained the mechanism of fasting and feasting on the molecular level. To answer the question about the benefits of intermittent fasting on human beings, there is no well known substitute in humans.

The Human Experience

Among the most consistent pioneers of intermittent fasting for weight loss is a nutritional researcher Dr. Krysta Varady from the University of Illinois in Chicago. Dr. Varady has published widely and deeply on the subject matter, and has summarized her findings in the book, Every Other Day Diet. Her book had a tagline of "4 weeks, two sizes, 12 pounds." Dr. Krysta Varady also ran a famous experiment before her conclusion.

In a magazine entitled JAMA that has been published recently, Dr. Varady reported on research that was carried out on one hundred obese people. These participants included 86 women and 14 men. The research was carried out for six months of weight loss phase which was followed by a six months' weight maintenance phase. In addition to the groups being randomized and professionally controlled, the trial lasted for one year, unlike other short-term studies.

Intermittent fasting is tricking your body and mind into consuming less food. Because you are losing weight, you are benefiting from the metabolism. This implies better compliance through mind tricks, although Dr. Varady concluded that the study did not produce superior adherence.

Nevertheless, there is much to admire in Dr. Varady here. She is a researcher who devoted her time and career to proving the clear benefits of intermittent fasting. She dared to run the definitive experiment. She also had the intellectual integrity to explain the facts, however inconvenient it looked. While conventional wisdom about dieting can't handle intermittent fasting and will go against it quite a bit, this type of eating pattern can make a big difference in weight loss, heart risks, and more. Let's look at some research behind intermittent fasting:

Alternate Day Fasting and Chronic Disease Prevention Study - 2007

The effects that were seen in how well intermittent fasting can work seems to vary between animals and humans. One exception to this is that the animal studies did show a decrease in blood pressure in those animals, but the human trials didn't seem to confirm this.

To the date of this study, the effects of alternate day fasting on cancer has only been done on animals. Many people believe that these same results would show up in humans who follow this method of fasting as well.

In terms of how alternate day fasting can help prevent and reduce type 2 diabetes, the results of the data from this study, and others have been inconsistent. It may have more to do with the diet plan the individual follows while they are on an intermittent fast. If you continue to eat junk while fasting, type 2 diabetes will not be cured.

Energy balance and reproductive dysfunction study conducted in 2013

For this study, three months old rats went through a period of fasting. They were deprived of food every other day for the entire day. Then on the non-fasting day, they were fed ad libitum.

This regimen ended up adversely affecting the reproduction in the rats by changing up the reproductive cycle in the female rats. This has been seen in humans as well. While women can also benefit from intermittent fasting, they need to be careful about the number of hours they enter a fasting state. Usually, it is recommended that women stick with a fourteen to sixteen hour fast to get the benefits but prevent issues associated with the disruption of their reproductive system.

Study on the potential benefits and harms of intermittent fasting - 2017

There were two studies done on healthy and overweight subjects. These individuals reported sustained hunger with this kind of fasting. They found that it was difficult for them to maintain daily living activities during restricted days of an alternate day fasting regimen.

However, in these two studies, when the participants changed to a 16: 8 version of intermittent fasting, these feelings of hunger tended to go away after just a few days.

A long-term study on the effects of the alternate day fasting

In the past, one of the most significant issues with intermittent fasting was that there weren't any long-term studies on it and how it could affect humans. Many of the studies done had been done on rats and other animals, and any human studies were reviews or only lasted a few weeks. But what about those who decided to use intermittent fasting for the long term and who wanted to know whether this diet plan was successful or not?

In one study published in JAMA Internal Medicine, people were studied for a whole year. For six of those months the individuals tried to lose weight and for the other six months they tried to maintain their weight loss. During the first six months, one-third of the subjects could eat what they wanted, one third had their three meals provided each day - which would take up 75 percent of their calorie needs - and the fasting group would alternate between a 500 and a 2500 calorie day.

By the end of this study, the subjects kept off about five to six percent of their weight, and they all had similar numbers when it came to fasting glucose, insulin resistance, cholesterol, heart rate, and blood pressure. However, the results for those in the fasting group may be skewed because 38% of the participants dropped out compared to the steady diet losing 29%, and the control group losing 26%. The averages include those who dropped out, so the weight loss may have been different if more people in the intermittent fasting group stayed with it longer.

So, this brings up the question about whether intermittent fasting was unique or not, or if you should go with a different type of diet. The subjects in this study were metabolically healthy obese women. Plus the food that these individuals ate was pretty standard and carb heavy. Many people who go on an actual intermittent fast will eat lower carb foods, which could help make the results more prominent.

Another thing to note is that this study only looked at one type of intermittent fasting. Many of the studies done on fasting will work with the 5:2 diet. This one has a little more time between fasts, while other options will have to do a mini-fast each day. Many claim that the shorter daily fasts are more effective when it comes to losing weight.

When you do go on an intermittent fasting diet, make sure that you also eat a healthy diet with healthy foods as well.

Harvard study shows how intermittent fasting may be the clue to anti-aging

Being able to manipulate the mitochondrial networks that are inside the cells, either by manipulating the genes or restricting your diet, can help you promote health and increase your lifespan. This is according to some new research that comes from the Harvard T.H. Chan School of Public Health.

Mitochondria, the structures in the cells that will produce energy, exist in networks that can change shape based on the demand for power from the body. Their ability to do this is going to go down with age, but the impact that this can have on cellular function and your metabolism were not understood before. With this study, researchers showed a causal link between dynamic changes in the shapes of mitochondria and longevity.

To test their theories, scientists worked with C. elegans. The mitochondrial networks that are inside a cell will usually switch between either fragmented or fused states. They only live for two weeks, which made it easier for the scientists to study how aging occurs at real time in their labs. These young networks were able to increase their lifespan by communicating with various organelles to help modulate the metabolism of fat.

While it has long been thought that dietary restrictions and intermittent fasting can help promote healthy aging, knowing why this all exists is a big step towards helping to harness the benefits and use them for our own needs. These findings from Harvard open up some new avenues in the search for strategies that can reduce a human's likelihood of developing diseases related to age as you get older.

The type of diet that works the best for this seems to be the 5:2 menu, but it is possible to see the results with any of the options that are out there for intermittent fasting. The way that we eat can affect how the genes in our body work, and even how the different parts of the cell behave together, and that can make such a difference in our longevity.

CHAPTER 4:

How To Start Intermittent Fasting

You've got everything you need now to get started losing weight, feeling better, and getting healthier using intermittent fasting.

Start by looking at your overall health as it currently stands. If you have any particular concerns (like diabetes or other medical and health issues), review your new intermittent fasting intentions with your doctor to be sure you're healthy enough to begin. Read through the vital information about each method of intermittent fasting. Consider your schedule, your lifestyle, and what you think might be most comfortable for you. You may consider trying a few different techniques before deciding on the one that will be most effective for you. Remember, with each technique, you can customize the fasting and eating hours to fit your preferences and schedule. The time of day of your fasting and when you eat is not what's important, so plan to break your fasts on days and during hours that will be convenient and most comfortable for you to stick to.

Once you've decided on a method, you're ready to start. Keep a journal or a log of the times and days you plan to fast, and when you'll be eating. Your body will adjust to your new pattern of eating, and your hunger signals will soon be all the reminder you need that it's time to break your most recent fasting cycle!

If you're perfectly happy with the amount of weight loss intermittent fasting provides you per week, you may decide not to add a daily exercise routine. Regular physical activity, including daily walks, may be enough for many people to lose weight while using intermittent fasting.

Transitioning to Intermittent Fasting

When you choose to start eating on an intermittent fasting cycle, it is always essential to make sure that you make the transition at a pace that is manageable by your body. Start slowly and pay attention to your symptoms. Do not attempt to set a time frame as to when you will move on to the next phase as this might result in you pushing yourself too quickly. Alternatively, you might find yourself waiting too long and wasting time. Instead, look to spend about three days on your current level of intermittent fasting without any challenging symptoms. Once you can go three consecutive days without experiencing headaches, constipation, exhaustion, or any other troubling symptoms, then you know you have acclimated to your new phase. Then, you can move on to your next one confidently.

Before you begin the intermittent fasting diet, take some time to learn what your natural eating pattern is. Spending just a few days discovering how you naturally eat can support you in understanding what you need to transition successfully. Even if you already have a reasonably good idea of what your natural eating pattern is, you should still spend a few days purposefully documenting it.

It is essential that you first work your way up to the 16:8 diet before moving into any other variation of the fast. In doing so, you teach your body to become used to fasting. Many people have claimed that doing their transition this way supported them in doing the 5:2 fast or the 24-hour weekly fast more successfully as it helped their body adapt more effectively. When you do this, you will help minimize your symptoms and support your ability to fast without shocking your body.

Knowing how to pay attention to your symptoms and giving your body what it needs is essential. When you take better care of yourself, your ability to successfully eat to this dietary style is improved. You also see better results from your diet because you are listening to your body's needs.

Pay attention to signs that you need to move slower, choose a less intense fasting cycle, or even run faster or choose a more intense one. When you know what you need and what you can handle, picking the right diet that is going to serve your health goals and keep you feeling great is much more comfortable.

When you choose healthier options, this will not only support you in feeling better during your fasting cycles, but it will also assist you in achieving your goals. Your healthier options will help you in experiencing higher energy levels, improved weight loss, increased muscle gain, and better overall health. As a result, your diet and eating cycles will both work together to help you achieve your goals faster and with greater sustainability.

Overeating sugar during your eating windows can result in a spike in your sugar levels. As you then move into the fasting window, the sugars are consumed but not replenished, so you suddenly experience a drop in your sugar levels. This spiking back and forth can be extremely unhealthy for your body. Furthermore, it can increase the number of unpleasant side effects that you experience on your diet.

To deal with this problem you should resume your healthy diet first. Then, if you feel that you want to, you might consider trying a less intense variation of the diet; such as the 12-hour fasting diet. Depending on the symptoms you had and the way you handled the transition, you might consider trying to increase your fasting windows slightly and seeing how that works for you. However, if you begin experiencing serious or damaging side effects again, you need to stop immediately, and you should refrain from eating this way.

CHAPTER 5:

Why Intermittent Fasting

Intermittent fasting is superior to virtually every other diet in many different ways. The nature of this diet is significantly different from the nature of other diets that people typically choose. Due to how this diet is structured, with a greater emphasis on when food is consumed versus what food is consumed, it provides more benefits than most traditional diets do.

The intermittent fasting diet is widely touted for its many health benefits, but it has some other benefits, too. For example, the diet is convenient. When you eat this way, you do not have to spend quite as much time cooking, eating, and cleaning up after. Instead of eating several meals per day, most intermittent fasters only eat one or two big meals and then a few snacks. Less time preparing and planning for meal times means that you can spend more time doing other things.

The other reason why the intermittent fasting diet is so popular is that you can still eat virtually anything you want on this diet. While this is not a reason to get silly with the desserts and go overboard on junk foods, you also do not have to worry about restricting yourself to just one cookie, or a 1/8" piece of cake at dessert. Instead, you can enjoy the full portion or a couple of cookies and have no worries about any repercussions that you may face.

The fact that you can continue eating how you want when you eat according to the intermittent fasting diet, makes this diet more sustainable than others. Other diets often require you to cut out certain things or reduce the types of food that you eat.

When you eat less, the calories you consume will decrease as well. When the levels of insulin decline, growth hormone increases along with an increase in norepinephrine, which helps the body break down stored fat to provide energy. There is an increase in your metabolic rate when you fast, which helps the body burn more calories. The effect of intermittent fasting is therefore two-fold.

The reduction in the level of food you consume reduces your overall calorie intake. Both of these conditions promote weight and fat loss.

Many people that have introduced Intermittent Fasting into their lifestyles have reported positive effects on their skin. Free radicals are produced by our bodies when we breathe. A decent and healthy level is subtle, as they stimulate repair. However, when our body produces more than it should, it can damage our cells, which is called oxidative stress. It is one of the factors for aging skin, wrinkles, and graying hair.

Another primary reason for inflammation is excessive free radicals in your body, resulting in cellular damage. When our cells' mitochondria (the powerhouse in our cells that give us energy) are damaged, they begin to release excessive free radicals. These, in turn, result in inflammation and DNA damage. All these problems vanish when you allow your body to be in a fasted state for extended hours.

The body is designed to operate effectively and efficiently when it runs on a lean diet. When it overheats, the body needs to spend a lot of its time digesting food and shuttling it to various areas and, when in excess, has to convert it to fat and store it.

To keep you in a state of rest, the shot of hormones places your mind in a relaxed state, and that reduces your mental acuity. It's primal in its design. Cave dwellers who needed to go out and hunt were given the extra boost in mental acuity and strength when they were hungry but turned sleepy and relaxed after a full meal. We, today, are no different. It has been researched and observed that intermittent fasting accelerates and prolongs the neural development in the brain.

It is now well documented that the oxidation leads to things like heart disease and stroke by leading to the hardening of arteries and blood vessels. Oxidative stress also alters gene expression and the regulation of tissue repair. That has a direct impact on how your cells age as you want them to be flexible and elastic. It results in better-looking skin and when you do lose weight, your skin will not sag because it is properly nourished.

Intermittent fasting improves LDL levels, which has a direct impact on cardiovascular health. This is done in two ways. First of all, it reduces the stress in your heart to keep working at digesting large quantities of food and storing energy in the fat cells. If you use what you take in, there is no need to put your heart through that stress. Ask anyone who is out of shape and on the larger side of life, how they feel after a meal – they will tell you they need to rest.

Fasting can lead to autophagy, which is a cellular process for removal of waste. This entails cells breaking down and metabolizing dysfunctional, broken proteins, which build up in cells over extended periods. During this autophagy, your body builds protection against several diseases like Alzheimer's disease and cancer.

The most common health problem that plagues humanity these days, apart from obesity, is diabetes. High blood sugar leads to insulin resistance in the body. Intermittent fasting helps to reduce blood sugar and therefore helps reduce insulin resistance in the body. If you opt for this diet, you can successfully reverse this condition.

One thing that many other diets do not accommodate for is eating out. Attempting to eat out when you are on a diet can be challenging. Choosing restaurants that serve foods that provide your needs or trying to educate your friends and family on what you can and cannot have, can be frustrating. It can cause people to avoid going out because they do not want to be a hassle to their loved ones or struggle to find something to eat at a restaurant. Intermittent fasting, on the other hand, allows you to eat out without much concern given to what you eat.

CHAPTER 6:

Different Methods Of Intermittent Fasting

While there are many methods for intermittent fasting, only a handful of them works well, and others work well for people in exceptional cases. Overall, the goal is to learn about each method, its strengths, and its weaknesses, and then to choose which is right for you, given the current stage of your life and what struggles you face at the moment.

Crescendo Method

The crescendo method of intermittent fasting is the one voted most productive for female-bodied practitioners. This method is well-known for its gentle approach to fasting, its caution, and awareness of hormonal balance, its ability to help you lose weight, and its gradual introduction (which works exceptionally well for people with inconsistent work or life schedules).

Through the crescendo method, the individual will fast 12 to 16 hours at a time for two or three days a week; not consecutive days. For instance, you might fast Sunday, normally eat Monday and Tuesday, fast Wednesday, usually eat Thursday, fast Friday, often eat on Saturday and repeat the pattern the next Sunday. During fast days, light cardio exercises or yoga can be practiced, but no intense workouts are allowed, due to the long hours involved in the fast. As needed, drink lots of water (with salt added if/when you get dizzy!) and coffee if you desire any energy boosts.

After two successful weeks of this pattern of fasting, additional days can be added, or the timing can be tweaked based on what's working and what isn't.

Lean-Gains Method (14:10)

The lean-gains method has several different incarnations on the web, but its fame comes from the fact that it helps shed fat while building it into muscle almost immediately. Through the lean-gains method, you'll find yourself able to shift all that fat to be muscle through a rigorous practice of fasting, eating right, and exercising.

Through this method, you fast anywhere from 14 to 16 hours and then spend the remaining 10 or 8 hours each day engaged in eating and exercise. This method, as opposed to the crescendo, features daily fasting and eating, rather than alternated days of eating versus not. Therefore, you don't have to be quite so cautious about extending the physical effort to exercise on the days you are fasting; because every day is a fasting day!

For the lean-gains method, start fasting for only 14 hours then work it up to 16 if you feel comfortable with it. Never forget to drink enough water and be careful about expending too much energy on exercise! Remember that you want to grow in health and potential through intermittent fasting. You'll certainly not want to lose any of that growth by forcing the process along.

16:8 Method

The 16:8 method of intermittent fasting is increasingly popular with practitioners of IF because it's often voted as the easiest one to enact. For some people especially, this method is the logical extension of the lean-gains way, except it places less focus on intense physical exercise that would accompany the fasting.

With the 16:8 methods of IF, you'll fast for 16 hours and then use the remaining 8-hour window to eat. Most people skip breakfast immediately upon waking and use their sleeping time to get that first 16 hours of fasting together. Others will stop eating earlier in the night and then breakfast will be their starting meal. Regardless, all the meals of the day will take place in the 8-hour eating window, which means you can probably fit three smaller meals into that time, but it can also mean that two meals might work better some days.

Overall, the 16:8 Method is a great one to start with, especially if you sleep ten or more hours each night. If you're not sure which method to begin with, try this one and then build up from it! Some people go from 16:8 to 20:4 while others use it as a diving board into alternate-day fasting. Try whatever works for you, but whatever you do, try!

20:4 Method

Stepping things up a notch from the 14:10 and 16:8 methods, the 20:4 Method is a tough one to master, for it is rather unforgiving.

People talk about this method of intermittent fasting as intense and highly restrictive, but they also say that the effects of living on this method are almost unparalleled with all other tactics.

For the 20:4 Method, you'll fast for 20 hours each day and squeeze all your meals, all your eating, and all your snacking into 4 hours. People who attempt 20:4 typically have two smaller meals or just one large meal and a few snacks during their 4-hour window to eat, and it is up to the individual which four hours of the day they devote to eating.

The trick for this method is to make sure you're not overeating or bingeing during those 4 hours. It is all-too-easy to get hungry during the 20-hour fast and have that feeling then propel you into intense and unrealistic hunger or meal sizes after the fasting period is over. Be careful if you try this method. If you're new to intermittent fasting, work your way up to this one gradually, and if you're working your way up already, only make the shift to 20:4 when you know you're ready. It would surely disappoint if all your progress with intermittent fasting got hijacked by one poorly thought-out goal with 20:4 methods.

12:12 Method

As another of the more natural ways of intermittent fasting, 12:12 approach is well-suited to beginning practitioners. Many people live out 12:12 method without any forethought simply because of their sleeping and eating schedule but turning 12:12 into a conscious practice can have just as many positive effects on your life as the more drastic 20:4 method claims.

According to a study conducted in the University of Alabama For this method, in particular, you fast for 12 hours and then enter a 12-hour eating window. It's not difficult whatsoever to get three small meals and several snacks, or two big meals and a snack into your day with this method. With 12:12, the standard meal timing works just fine.

Ultimately, this method is a great one to start with, for a lot of variation can be built into this scheduling when you're ready to make things more interesting. Effortlessly and without much effort, 12:12 can become 14:10 or even 16:8, and in seemingly no time, you can find yourself trying alternate-day or crescendo methods, too. Start with what's normal for you, and this method might be exactly that!

5:2 Method

When it comes to the intermittent fasting methods that have several hours each day set aside to fast and the lingering hours set aside to eat, something gets lost in translation. Some people come to intermittent fasting with aims at significant lifestyle changes, or with hopes of experiencing whole new timing and relationships to food. In that case, these individuals might prefer 5:2 Method.

Like the crescendo method, 5:2 goes back to several days "on" and several days a week "off" when it comes to fasting. More specifically, this method of IF (being more extreme than any others we've looked at so far) involves a severe restriction of caloric intake for two days a week and regular feeding the remaining five days. On the two restricted-intake days, the practitioner is only allowed 500 calories per day to maintain and actualize the goals of the fast.

If you're having trouble making 5:2 method work, try a different style of intermittent fasting altogether. It could be that this strange on-and-off method doesn't suit your lifestyle, and there are enough other options that there's bound to be something that works just right for you.

Eat-Stop-Eat (24 Hour) Method

This method of fasting is incredibly similar to the crescendo method. The only discernable difference is that there's no anticipation of increasing (of "crescendo-ing") into a more intense fasting pattern with time. For the eat-stop-eat method, you decide which days you want to take off from eating, and then you run with it until you've lost that weight and then you keep running with the lifestyle for good because you won't be able to imagine life without it.

The eat-stop-eat method involves one to two days a week being 100% oriented towards fasting, with the other five to six days concerning "business as normal." The one or two days spent fasting are then full 24-hour days spent without eating anything at all. During these days, of course, water and coffee are still okay to drink. In fact, anything is still acceptable to drink during fasting periods as long as it's not too thick, like a smoothie or protein shake. However, no food items can be consumed whatsoever. Exercise is also frowned upon on those fasting days but see what your body can handle before you decide how that should all work out.

Some people might start thinking they're using the crescendo method but end up sticking with eat-stop-eat. The two are so similar. Furthermore, some others work up to the eat-stop-eat method from 14:10 or 16:8 ways. It could be that these individuals tried the daily fast window technique and wanted something more intense. This method qualifies!

Alternate-Day Method

The alternate-day method is admittedly a little confusing, but the reason it could be so complicated could come, in part, from how much wiggle room it provides for the practitioner. This method is excellent for people who don't have a consistent schedule or any sense of one, and it is therefore incredibly forgiving for those who don't quite have everything together for themselves yet.

When it comes down to it, alternate-day intermittent fasting is really up to you. You should try to fast every other day, but it doesn't have to be that precise. Similarly, with the crescendo method, as long as you fast two to three days a week, with a break day or two in between each fasting day, you're set! Then, you'll want to eat regularly for three or four days out of each week, and when you encounter a fasting day, you don't even need to completely fast! All you need to do on these days is restrict your caloric intake to 20-25% of your standard intake (~500 calories total, each day).

Alternate-day fasting is a reliable place to start from, primarily if you work a varying schedule or still have yet to get used to a consistent one. If you want to make things more intense from this starting point, the alternate-day method can quickly become the eat-stop-eat method, the crescendo method, or the 5:2 method. Essentially, this method is a great place to begin.

The Warrior Method

The warrior method is incredibly similar to the 20:4 method, but with one significant philosophical difference, which makes this method all that much more interesting. The warrior method takes as its philosophical base the experience of the hunter/gatherer ancestors we evolved from. It's as if this method looks back at the origins of intermittent fasting and tries to make its example as historically accurate as possible.

In sum, warrior method involves fasting for 20 hours a day (although you can have one cup of raw, fresh fruit and vegetables dispersed throughout that 20 hours) and then eating one large meal during the 4-hour feeding window. Just like the warrior coming home from the hunt, the individual practicing warrior method will spend most of the day working (i.e., the fast lasts all day). Only to come home and focus on one large meal (i.e., the 4-hour eating window would always take place during the evening), from which the body can then extract all its necessary nutrients and proteins for energy, alertness, and fat burning.

Warrior method is the logical extension of 20:4 method when you want to take things up a notch of intensity (or of philosophical rigor). It can also be scaled back to 16:8 or 14:10 quickly, if you notice things just aren't working with this method for you. The most significant danger of warrior method is overeating during that one meal.

Spontaneous Skipping Method

As the purposefully least-organized method of the bunch, the automatic skipping method leaves most of the definition and planning to the individual. There's no natural division of time between fasting and feeding. There's no delineating of how much time needs to be spent on what. There are no standards for this plan whatsoever. The individual determines all this planning for him or herself.

Skip breakfast and your second snack one day, skip lunch and dinner the next (in favor of a bedtime snack), and then skip breakfast again the day after. Skip meals based on what's convenient for you, too!

If you're someone who has trouble defining a daily schedule, someone who balks at routine, or works increasingly varying shifts at work; this intermittent fasting method is probably perfect for you. Try this one out to start or try it after you've realized some of the more "structured" ways don't work, based on your lifestyle.

Regardless of how you do it, try it! Even if you're not fully functioning at intermittent fasting quite yet, dip your toes in the water! Skip a meal here and there, and I promise, your body will thank you for it.

CHAPTER 7:

Why 16:8 Intermittent Fasting Method Is The Best

Intermittent fasting techniques, including the 16:8 method, are most commonly used to assist in weight loss by the general population. The technique has been tried by thousands of people and also scientifically proven to be a helpful resource in reducing body fat and improving body composition. Weight loss is often considered the number one reason why people opt for a diet and program that utilizes intermittent fasting. Studies conducted in different areas of the world found that intermittent fasting is efficient for weight loss.

While a reduction in body fat is definitely one of the best advantages to be mentioned in terms of intermittent fasting, there are more advantages that people gain when they decide that they are going to follow this type of program – especially if they truly commit to it and can implement self-control that ensures they do not give in to cravings.

Intermittent fasting is known to assist in improving your body composition as well; a series of features including your body fat percentage and lean muscle mass primarily. A program that utilizes intermittent fasting, along with an appropriate diet plan, will bring down your body fat percentage, and push up your lean muscle mass at the same time.

It is also important to note the benefits that are associated with weight loss for people with an excessive amount of fat distributed throughout their body. Since overweight and obesity are linked to so many chronic diseases that can truly make your life dreadful, losing even small amounts of weight can drastically reduce your risk of these diseases.

When you develop type 2 diabetes, you become predisposed to many additional risks and complications. Type 2 diabetes can cause severe complications that may not only lead to disability but also become life-threatening. This disease can also affect all of the body's most essential organs, including the heart, and can damage various tissues, such as nerves, throughout the body.

In addition to assisting in reducing body weight and bringing down the risks associated with obesity, intermittent fasting has many other benefits that are also worth mentioning. Through intermittent fasting, cellular changes may occur in the body. This can lead to levels of human growth hormones rising by as much as 500%. This leads to a faster rate of fat burning while also producing an increase in muscle mass.

This means that cells in the body become more efficient in performing their specialized functions.

Furthermore, following an intermittent fasting plan can also help to reduce levels of inflammation within the human body, as well as help to fight against oxidative stress. Both of these factors are known to contribute to numerous chronic diseases significantly and can cause specific molecules to become damaged, which can inhibit their functionality within the body.

The 16:8 method is one of the easiest to follow and most comfortable to understand, which is why many beginners choose it. Of course, it doesn't suit everyone, and because one size doesn't fit all, it might be that some people switch to a different method after a short amount of time. That's fine, and that might be something you want to think about. We're going to cover some alternative methods a little later in the book, so always bear in mind that if you find the 16:8 method isn't working as well as you want it to, for you, then there are other alternatives.

For the most part, however, the 16:8 Method, or Lean Gains, is very successful for many, and it is a method which encourages healthy eating without rules and regulations in terms of restrictions. There are no massive changes to lifestyle, which is something which many people struggle with when they try a different eating routine, e.g. the Keto Diet, Atkins, Paleo, etc. These all come with a lot of rules and regulations, and there are lists of what you can and can't eat, and how it should be prepared. This can overwhelm many a beginner and cause them to rebel against it and say: 'no thanks!' The 16:8 method and many other intermittent fasting methods don't come with those rules attached.

The other plus point is that the 16:8 Method doesn't have to bother your social life. Most people want to head out with friends or their partner for dinner on occasion, or perhaps out for a few drinks, but this can be very difficult when following a low calorie or fad diet. With the 16:8 Method, all you need to do is ensure that you schedule the get-together for your eating window. This might be more difficult if you're starting your eating window early and finishing early, but you can always meet up for lunch instead of dinner! There aren't restrictions on what you can eat, but in most restaurants, you can still make healthy choices on the regular menu. If your eating window finishes a little later, that means you have more scope in terms of time.

Let's sum up the main reasons why most beginners opt for the 16:8 Method.

• It's easy to follow and doesn't require any counting, weighing, or monitoring

• You can alter your eating time according to your needs

• You can set much of your fasting period to coincide with your sleeping period, so you don't notice it quite so much

• The eating method doesn't need to interfere with your social life too much at all

• You are not restricted on what you can eat, provided you make sensible, generally healthy choices

• It doesn't feel like a diet, it feels more like a new lifestyle with timings, rather than food you can and can't eat

• You can still have calorie-free drinks, water, and unsweetened, black tea or coffee during your fast

• You won't notice hunger quite so much with this type of eating plan, as there are no extremely long fasts involved

CHAPTER 8:

The 16/8 Method-Everyday Method

We've mentioned that there are many different types of intermittent fasting, and some do ask you to fast for 24 hours, several times a week. The 16:8 method differs because there are no long and arduous fasts, you fast for 16 hours every day, and eat regularly for 8 hours.

Now, that sounds like a lot - 16 hours, but you are going to be sleeping for most of it! You see, you can move the fasting period to suit your needs. We'll talk about how to follow the method in more detail shortly, but a good example is someone who needs to eat breakfast versus someone who doesn't specifically want to eat early in the mornings. We're all different, but most of us fall into one of these two categories. You might wake up starving hungry and need breakfast; otherwise, you can't focus, or you might wake up and need a coffee, and you feel a little sick if you eat straight away. There are two ways you can manage this, to give you an example of what the 16:8 method looks like.

If you need breakfast, you can eat it as soon as you wake up, kick-starting your 8-hour eating period. If you wake up at 8:00am, you have breakfast at 8.30am, then that means you need to finish eating by 4.30pm. You might go to bed at 10 pm, which means you're only consciously fasting 5½ hours. As you can see, it's not as horrendous as it sounds, and you can drink water, non-calorie containing drinks, and unsweetened, black tea or coffee during your fasting times too. It's highly recommended that you drink plenty of water anyway because dehydration is not something you want to play Russian roulette with!

The other scenario is that you are someone who doesn't want to eat when they wake up. In that case, you can get up, get dressed, have a black, unsweetened coffee, and you can skip breakfast, starting your eating window at lunchtime. So, for instance, you would start eating at noon. This means you can eat freely until 8:00pm. You would then perhaps sleep at 10 pm, which means you're effectively not consciously fasting too much! This is why the 16:8 Method is so popular.

Of course, during your 8-hour eating window, you need to be mindful of what you're eating. If you cram those 8 hours full of crisps and chocolate, then you're going to eat far more calories than you should in a 24-hours day. If however, you're mindful of what you eat, not mainly being restrictive, but merely thinking more along the lines of health, you'll be full and satisfied by the end of your eating window and ready for your fast. This means you will lose weight quite quickly and grab the overall benefits of intermittent fasting too.

How to Follow The 16:8 Method

The 16:8 Method is very flexible, and that means you can choose your own specific 8-hour eating window, according to your day. You might work shifts, and that means you sleep at different times. What you should do in that case is pick an 8-hour window which is when you are mostly awake. Obviously!

For example, if you are working nights and you are sleeping between the hours of 10:00am and 6:00pm, that means you can eat from 6:00pm until 2:00am. You would then probably be working until the following morning when you would head off to sleep, but you could drink coffee (unsweetened and black) to keep you going also, and plenty of water. This might not work for you, so you could think about shifting your pattern and starting it later, perhaps if you don't feel like eating the moment you open your eyes. You could then choose an eating window of 9:00pm and eat freely until 5:00am.

It's not only about when you can eat, but it's also about what you eat too. While there are no restrictions and no lists of foods you must eat and foods you shouldn't, always remember that if you suddenly pile a huge breakfast or lunch on your plate after fasting, you're going to end up with stomach ache. That could mean that you end up eating too many calories within your eating window and actually put weight on, or you end up with stomach disturbances for the rest of your eating window, don't get enough fuel during that time because your stomach is so bloated you can't bear to eat, and then you're hungry during your fasting time. It's about choosing carefully, which we'll talk about a little more shortly.

So, how many calories should you eat? A standard calorie amount to maintain weight is 2500 calories per day for a man. This does depend on the height, current weight, and metabolism of the person, and is only an average, healthy amount. If you want more solid guidelines on your specific circumstances, speak to your doctor, who will be able to give you a calorie aim plan tailored to your needs.

Within that calorie amount, you should make sure that you get a proper, varied diet. That means proteins, carbs, fats, vitamins, and minerals. Again, we're going to cover what you can and can't eat, loosely because there are no rules, shortly, but varied is the way to go. Ironically, this will also help you enjoy your new lifestyle more, because you're not bored and eating the same things all the time. This is a pitfall many people suffer from regular low-calorie diets; the change is so restrictive that they end up eating the same thing day in, day out, and over time they get so bored and rebel against it. This usually ends in a binge day, which causes extreme guilt and then leads them to throw the diet in the bin and go back to eating whatever they want.

While following the 16:8 Method, you should also make sure that you drink plenty of water throughout the day, whether fasting or eating. This ensures that you don't become dehydrated and will also aid in digestion. Besides, you should also exercise too!

Now, there are no rules to say that you must exercise while following an intermittent fasting routine, but it will help you lose weight faster, and it will help with your general health and wellbeing. Exercise is fantastic on so many levels, not least helping to build lean muscle, which also boosts your ability to burn fat as an energy source. Exercise is also known to help with mental health issues, such as anxiety and depression, as well as stress. We all live stressful lives, and a little exercise can sometimes be enough to reduce it to extremely manageable levels. Aside from anything else, training can be a friendly and fun activity!

⬚ Eat for 8 hours per day, consecutively - you cannot break these hours up, they must be observed as one block of time

⬚ Fast for 16 hours per day, again, this needs to be done consecutively

⬚ You can choose when you take your 8-hour eating block, but it's a good idea to stick to the same times every day, so your body gets into a routine

⬚ Your fasting times should coincide with sleeping, to cut down on the amount of conscious fasting

⬚ Do not be afraid to miss breakfast, in this eating routine; there is no 'important meal of the day,' there is simply a vital eating window

⬚ You can drink unsweetened, black tea and coffee, water, and other non-calorie containing drinks freely throughout your eating and fasting times, and you should undoubtedly consume enough water throughout the day to ensure you don't become dehydrated

☐ During your eating period, you should spread your meals out carefully, so you don't 'binge' when you initially break your fast. This will only lead to stomach aches and other unpleasant gastric symptoms!

☐ Choose healthy meals as much as possible, but there are no restrictions on what you can eat. If you go unhealthy, however, remember that you're not going to create the calorie deficit required for weight loss

☐ Whilst you don't need to count calories while following the 16:8 Method, it's worth bearing the standard calorie amounts in mind, which is 2500 for a man and 2000 for a woman, every day, as an average.

☐ Never be tempted to cut down your eating window or to restrict your calorie amount beneath the average - this will lead to extreme hunger and even borderline starvation if you refuse to eat. Remember, fasting is not starving!

What You Can and Can't Eat

Again, there are no rules on what you can eat and what you can't eat, it's a free choice when following the 16:8 diet.

The idea is to create that calorie deficit during the full 24-hour span. You do this by ensuring that you fast and eat for the correct ratios of time, e.g., 8 hours eating and 16 hours fasting, and that during your eating times you stick to healthy options as much as possible. You will feel infinitely better as a result also.

If you want a few ideas on some of the healthiest foods you can incorporate into your day generally, check out the list below.

• Eggs - Make sure you eat the yolk because this contains the vitamins and protein!

• Leafy greens - We're talking about things like spinach, collards, Kale, and Swiss chards to name a few, and these are packed with fiber and low in calories too.

• Oily and fatty fish, such as salmon - Salmon is a fish which will keep you feeling full, but it's also high in omega three fatty acids which are ideal for boosting brain health, reducing inflammation, and generally helping with weight loss too. If salmon isn't your bag, try mackerel, trout, herring, and sardines instead.

• Cruciferous vegetables - In this case, you need to look toward Brussels sprout, broccoli, cabbage, and cauliflower. Again, these types of plants contain a high fiber amount which helps you feel fuller for longer, but also have cancer-fighting attributes.

• Lean meats - Stick to beef and chicken for the best options, but make sure that you go for the leanest cuts possible. You'll get a good protein boost here, but you can also make all manner of delicious dishes with both types of meat!

• Boiled potatoes - You might think that potatoes are rotten for you, and in most cases, they are, especially if you fry them, but boiled potatoes are a good choice, especially if you lack in

potassium. They are also very filling.

• Tuna - This is a different type of fish to the oily fish we mentioned earlier, and it's low in fat, but high in protein. Go for tuna, which is canned containing water and not oil for the healthiest option. Pile it onto a jacket potato for a delicious and healthy meal!

• Beans and other types of legumes - These are the staple of any healthy diet and are super filling too. We're talking about things like kidney beans, lentils and black beans here, and they're high in fiber and protein.

• Cottage cheese - If you're a cheese fan, there's no reason to deny yourself, but most cheeses are quite high in fat. In that case, why not opt for cottage cheese instead? This is high in protein and quite filling, but low in calories.

• Avocados - This fad food of the moment is very healthy and great for boosting your brain power! Mash it up on some toast for a great breakfast packed with potassium and plenty of fiber.

• Nuts - Instead of snacking on chocolate and crisps, why not snack on nuts? You'll get significant amounts of healthy fats, as well as fiber and protein, and they're filling too. Don't eat too many however, as they can be high in calories if you overindulge.

• Whole grains - Everyone knows that whole grains are packed with fiber and therefore keep you fuller for longer, so this is the ideal choice for anyone who is trying intermittent fasting. Try quinoa,

brown rice, and oats to get you started.

• Fruits - Not all fruits are healthy, but they're certainly a better option than chocolate and crisps! You'll also get a plethora of different vitamins and minerals, as well as a boost of antioxidants into your diet - ideal for your immune system.

• Seeds - Again, just like nuts, seeds make a great snack, and they can be sprinkled on many foods, such as yogurt and porridge. Try chia seeds for a high fiber treat, while being low calorie at the same time.

• Coconut oil and extra virgin olive oil - You will no doubt have heard of the wonders of coconut oil, and this is a very healthy oil to try cooking with. Coconut oil is made up of something called medium chain triglycerides, and whilst you might panic at the word triglycerides, these are actually the healthy type! If you want to go for something deficient in calories; however, then you can't beat extra virgin olive oil.

• Yogurt - Perfect for a gut health boost, yogurt is your friend because it will keep you full and it also has probiotic content, provided you go for products which say 'live and active cultures' on the pot. Avoid the overly sugary yogurt treats and anything which says 'low fat' usually isn't as positive as it sounds!

We're going to run you through some recipes a little later in the book, so you can see how easy healthy eating can be, and how satisfying too.

What shouldn't you eat?

There is nothing that is off limits, but it's about how much of it you eat. Remember, one of the reasons why intermittent fasting is so popular is because it doesn't wag its finger at you when you grab a chocolate bar once in a while. You don't have to feel guilty because you gave in to a burger craving once in a week, provided you know that moderation has to stand in the middle of it all.

What is moderation exactly? It knows when to stop and knowing what is enough and what is too much. For instance, enjoying pizza in moderation could mean having a couple of slices of pizza once a week. You still get to enjoy what you like, but you don't have it all the time. Similarly, moderation is stopping at two glasses of wine, rather than drinking the bottle. It means you still get what you want, but you don't go OTT.

To lose weight, you must ingest fewer calories than your body uses for all of its functions during a given time window. The interesting thing about eating in an 8-hour window is: there is only so much that you can eat before you feel full. This means it is important to eat according to your expected energy expenditure and activity levels. Below, is an example of a menu you can use to start the 16/8 Intermittent Fast.

From an exercise standpoint, try to fast through the time when you usually exercise. While you fast, you can exercise in the morning right when you wake up, or just before lunchtime. The key is to

exercise fasted, keeping your body in a Ketogenic state, so you are burning fat for fuel rather than sugars or simple carbohydrates.

CHAPTER 9:

What Are Macronutrients

It's pretty simple, macronutrients/macros are the proteins, carbohydrates and fats in the number of grams that is in your daily caloric intake. Every gram of protein, carbohydrate and fat has a calorie count:

Protein: 1g= 4 calories

Fat: 1g= 9 calories

Carbohydrate: 1g=4 calories

Proteins

Protein is the most important macronutrient while dieting. Amino acid availability is directly proportional to protein synthesis/muscle building. Protein can help maintain muscle while in a caloric deficit because it increases protein synthesis. It can also help build muscle while in a caloric surplus for the same reason.

Carbohydrates

Carbohydrates or "carbs" have gotten a bad name over the last couple of decades. This is largely due to the low-carb diet craze. But, if you have tried a low-carb diet, then you have probably found yourself both losing weight and losing your energy level. That is because of how the body uses carbohydrates.

Fats

If you are not getting enough fats, then you can experience hormonal imbalance. It can cause some hormone levels to decrease. This decrease in hormone levels can have adverse effects on your overall health.

You are going to see a pattern here. Fats can also be detrimental to your health in large quantities. Since fats are calorically dense, if you eat too much fats, then your body will store the excess as body fat. This is why moderation is in order. You need to strike a balance between eating enough fats to ensure proper hormone function but not so much that your body fat percentage increases.

What is the proper balance? This is the million-dollar question. It is also the thing that the majority of people don't know. It is really not that hard. I recommend that you keep your intake of fats between 15% and 30% of your total caloric intake.

You now have a basic understanding of the three macronutrients. This is the start of your journey towards controlling your weight. The next step is to understand how to calculate your macros.

How to calculate your macros?

In order to calculate your macros, you will need to use a

combination of proteins, fats and carbohydrates. As mentioned above each of the 3 macronutrients contains a certain energy value(calories) Protein: 1g= 4 kcal calories, Fat: 1g= 9 kcal calories, and Carbohydrate: 1g=4 kcal calories

The key is not to cut any one thing out of your diet completely. It is to learn how everything affects your body and then use moderation to control your intake. This helps to ensure that your body is able to work at its peak performance level.

For most areas of the world, the energy value of a food is measured for 100g of product. That means that the energy value of a food is determined by the macronutrients it contains in 100g.

For Instance: 100g of Zucchini muffin contains the following macronutrients - 9g

protein, 3g fats, and about 50g of carbs. The energy contained in 100g of the Zucchini muffin would therefore be:

9g protein x 4 kcal + 3g fats x 9 kcal + 50g carbs x 4 kcal = 263 kcal.

The Micronutrients

These are the partners of macronutrients, and it is essential to balance your macros with micronutrients to aid in your overall health. Micronutrients are the vitamins and minerals that are contained in your food. These micronutrients will help you control your emotions more easily; hormones produced by the body in a section of the brain called the amygdala are more balanced. For example, Vitamin B complex found in your local drug store will help you reduce anxiety and stress. Micronutrients additionally are essential to the mitochondrial energy chain. The mitochondria of the cells is what change the fatty acids from fats and the glucose from protein and carbohydrates in the food that we eat into cellular energy. The producing of this cellular energy is dependent upon multiple cofactors and numerous enzymatic transformations. Once the respective fuels, glucose or fatty acids, enter the mitochondria, there are multiple different vitamins, minerals, and amino acids which are necessary to convert them into ATP (adenosine triphosphate). Some of these micronutrients are manganese, magnesium, iron, B6, B12, and coenzymeQ10.

Mitochondrial energy is essential for proper liver function to help detoxify the many chemicals in the air, water, and food; and is necessary for ongoing cellular repair and maintenance. It is also required to get rid of metabolic waste from the brain. Without necessary micronutrients, cell membranes, which consist of about 80% fat, cannot do their functions. Adequate fatty acid intake is critical for good brain function. Cell membranes take in nutrients to produce energy, they maintain and repair as well as dispose of the cellular waste, take in the good and get rid of the bad. For example, glutamate, a primary stimulatory neurotransmitter, is dependent upon calcium, magnesium, and zinc to be adequate levels to be absorbed into the neuron. In essence, it has a triple lock system: one for the zinc, one for the calcium, and one for the glutamate.

For everyone in general, I suggest that they take multivitamins. The recommended dosages are regulated by the FDA and are on each bottle of tablets. Some vitamins are specifically formulated for women, for men, for pregnant women, for elderly women and men, and for children.

Note the vital effects of these vitamins and minerals:

▢ **Vitamin A** - This aids in your vision, bone growth, and metabolism.

▢ **Vitamin B1 (Thiamine)** - Thiamine helps you to break down those carbohydrates you consume.

▢ **Vitamin B2 (Riboflavin)** - This vitamin helps you break down your proteins, fats, and carbohydrates as well.

▢ **Vitamin B7 (Biotin)** - Biotin is essential in the conversion of carbohydrates into glucose, which is used for your energy. The best source for this is a multivitamin tablet.

▢ **Vitamin B9** - Folate is converted by the drug industry into its more usable form, FOLIC ACID. It is not produced by the body, but can be consumed in pill form. Some foods contain folate like lentils and asparagus. It is an aid to pregnant women.

▢ **Vitamin C** - The antioxidants available in Vitamin C help you fight off colds, other diseases, and prevent the occurrence of free

⊡ radicals (spoken about often in association with preventing cancer).

⊡ **Vitamin D** - Also called "Sunshine Vitamin", is produced by your body in the presence of natural sunlight. It is an important vitamin for menopausal women, in combination with calcium. Vitamin D aids in the breakdown of Calcium needed to increase bone strength.

⊡ **Vitamin E** - This is another crucial antioxidant vital in maintaining one's immune system at an optimal level. It also helps you recover from intensive workout routines by flushing out the built-up lactic acid in your muscle groups.

⊡ **Vitamin F** - These are important fatty acids. Only one of them (linoleic acid) is manufactured by your body. It is formed into lipids in cell membranes and the like. The other fatty acids have to be obtained outside of the body. Omega 3 fatty acid, praised heavily by nutritionists, is one of them. It is found in fish.

⊡ **Vitamin B5** is used to treat acne, allergies, baldness and heart failure. It is responsible for hormone production and cell division. Vitamin B5 is also used to cure low blood pressure, headache and muscle dystrophy. The best sources are mushrooms, avocado, potato, yogurt, turkey and broccoli.

⊡ **Vitamin B6** is used to cure skin rashes, fatigue and mood changes. It is responsible for the production of serotonin and adrenaline. Vitamin B6 is also responsible for the formation of a protective layer around the nerve cell. It is known that vitamin B6 can create various enzymes that are required for cell metabolism. The best sources are tuna, beef, turkey, salmon, banana and spinach.

 Vitamin B12 is used to cure heart failure, male infertility, osteoporosis, allergies and sleep disorders. Scientists believe it can drastically slow down the aging process. The best sources are meat, cheese, milk and eggs.

 You probably noticed that B vitamins have similar effects and many are found in the same sources. That is a great thing because you can obtain several B vitamins from the same source and save time and effort.

 Vitamin K. Vitamin K is one of the fat-soluble vitamins. Vitamin K is very important compound because of its role in the blood clotting process. The name is derived from the German word "koagulation ", which means blood clotting. People believe that blood clotting is always bad, but in many cases it is very important for our blood to clot. For example, blood clots form to stop bleeding when our skin gets cut or punctured.

How to Determine Your Ideal Macro Formula?

Before you start, please note that there is no sure-fire formula for this calculation. Among the different schools of thought, there is controversy. People are different and also have varying needs. Find what works for your body. Don't overlook the fact that you know yourself better than anyone else! Trust yourself when working out

your personal Macro formula!

The Easy Method

Check out the nutrition facts on the foods you eat. Anything packaged including meat is labeled in grams. Produce usually is not. For fruits and vegetables in the produce aisle, simply look it up on the internet.

For Weight Loss:

Daily formula -- 45% protein, 20% carbohydrates, 35% fats

For Body Building:

Daily formula -- 30% protein, 50% carbohydrates, 20% fats

Note that the male formula runs about 10% higher than the female formula, with the exception of carbohydrate intake. That is because men build larger muscles than women genetically.

The Challenging Method

Clinical studies have indicated that this more numerical method often works better for weight loss. I would recommend it for those who are quite obese and really, really need to lose weight, or for those who are very weak and need to build up their muscles. Time to do some math!

Here's how it's done:

Sedentary Job and Lifestyle

No offense intended, folks! Some of you spend most of your day inputting data into your computer. For that, you get paid. Where would we be without you?

Multiply your body weight in pounds by 11.

Moderately Active Job and Lifestyle

This means that you spend most of your workday walking and moving about. In addition, you work out at least 2 times per week.

Multiply your body weight in pounds by 12.

Active Job and Lifestyle

Your job requires movement other than just walking about and you exercise at least 3 times per week. This might apply to a housecleaner or handyman. That's enough to work up a sweat! You burn fat when that happens, and you know you do, don't you?

Multiply your body weight in pounds by 13.

Very Active Job and Lifestyle

This might be a construction worker, for example. Haven't you seen overweight construction workers, too? It seems ludicrous. The reason they are overweight is because they do not have their macros in balance! That is why this eating technique is extremely effective.

Multiply your body weight in pounds by 14.

NOW, WRITE DOWN THAT NUMBER! That is the total number of calories you would need per day depending on the levels of activity for your job and lifestyle.

Calculate Your Target Caloric Formula:

Take the number you worked out above. That is how many calories you need per day. Example: A 150-pound woman of average height who works at a sedentary job and does little exercise would need 150 x 11 = 1,650 total calories per day.

Then calculate in more detail, the calories of protein, fats and carbs.

Calories of Protein You Need per Day

The number of grams you need is your actual bodyweight in pounds. Write that down. Of course, you will remember that number, anyway. Example: A lovely 150-pound lady of average height wants to lose weight. She would need 150 grams protein per day.

Determine your protein calories. There are 4 calories per gram in protein. For our lady, that would be 150 x 4 = 600 calories protein.

Calories of Fats You Need per Day

Multiply your body weight by 0.5. Example: Our 150-pound woman would need: 150 x 0.5 = 75 grams. Is she smiling, I wonder?

Calories of Carbohydrates You Need per Day

Here's where it gets tricky...those troublesome carbohydrates! Yes, by all means, use a calculator, unless you are a true pioneer!

Now add the 2 numbers (proteins + fat) together and subtract the answer from the ideal number of calories your need per day. Example: Our woman would use the following calculations:

600 calories of protein + 675 calories of fat = 1,275 calories of protein + fat

Then MINUS that number from the total calories per day.

1,650 total number of daily calories - 1,275 protein + fat calories

= 375 calories of carbohydrates

Convert the carbohydrate calories into grams. There are 4 calories per gram of carbs, so divide:

375 ÷ 4 = 93.75 rounded down to 93 grams of carbohydrates needed

Calculate Your Macros Formula:

Daily Macros Formula: number of grams of proteins, number of grams of fat, number of grams of carbohydrates. For our 150-pound woman that would be:

150 g proteins, 75 g fat, 93 g carbohydrates

Keep track of your weight. If you aren't showing some progress in a

week, decrease all your macronutrients. Adjust your intake each week as your weight changes. You may even need to recalculate your macros as you go through the process. It is a tedious task, but you are worth the effort. How you look and feel is an important factor in bolstering your sense of self-esteem.

The clinical studies have shown that the most successful Macro dieters use digital scales to calculate their calories and grams. If you are meticulous, use one, or at least try. It will bring about more certain results.

How to Track Macronutrient Ratios?

Now that you know what your calorie requirements are for each day and you have worked out your macronutrient ratios, it is time to work out how many grams of each of the three nutrients you need. To do this, multiply your total calorie intake per day by each of the nutrition percentages in your ratio. The most important part now is to track every gram that you eat. You can either download a mobile App that will do it for you or you need to write down everything that you eat and how many grams of each of the macronutrients it contains.

Get into the habit of looking at the labels on everything and write down the grams of each of the nutrients. If there is no food label, you will need to use an app or look up the exact nutritional facts on the Internet. You will also need to write down exactly how much of each specific food you consume. If the food is processed, you can eat a set

amount and use the labels on the packaging to work out your grams. If, however, you are using whole natural foods, you must measure your portions carefully and work out your grams from that.

As you write everything down, pay close attention to your percentages and ratios through the course of the day. That way you can make any adjustments that are needed, ensuring that your final meal of each day has the right percentages to make your ratio up to 100%. If you cannot hit your percentages exactly, do not worry because the cumulative effect is just as important.

Along with methods of tracking your macro intake, several different strategies are common in the flexible dieting world.

Basic Calorie Tracking

This method is used in tons of different diet plans including the ever-popular Weight Watchers and even, in a sense, Flexible Dieting.

Following the basic calorie tracking method of weight loss, gain, or maintaining means you simply count your daily calorie intake from all foods and nutrients. This is only slightly different from tracking Macros, as it includes calories from all sources of food and not just proteins, carbohydrates, and fats you ingest.

Make sure you are keeping a weight loss journal on you at all times. This way you can write down what you ate and how many calories you consumed. Also, it is a good idea to write down in the beginning of your weight loss journal, how many pounds you would like to

lose. Make sure you write down all of your goals for each week or month. Weigh yourself once a week and write down how much the scale says and compare the weight loss from the previous week.

For women the most common calorie intake is 1,200 calories per day, but it still depends on your age, height, and how active you are. For example; if you are semi-active, between the ages of 30-50, then you should consume no more than 1,800 calories per day when trying to lose weight. If you aren't very active, then try to stick to the 1,200 calorie intake per day.

For men the calorie intake should be 16 calories per pound of body weight if you exercise regularly, 13 calories per pound if you workout moderately, and 11 calories per pound if you are over the age of 50 and do not exercise frequently. So, multiply the calories per weight to figure out how many calories you should be consuming everyday.

Food items with a low caloric density contain more water, more fibers and relatively less calories than richer options. Above all, they present the great advantage to make you feel full for a long time.

In fact, those low-caloric-density foods unlock less energy per gram of food. It is therefore possible to eat bigger quantities of them without putting on extra weight. Fruits, vegetables, soups, stews... all of them are part of that family.

The BNF recommends to base one's diet on low-caloric-density food (food that contains less than 1.5 calories per gram).

Whether you go for the Caloric Density approach or just want to learn more about what you eat, calorie control is key when trying to lead a healthier life. Re-learning to eat the right amounts of the right food can be both confusing and challenging. As I believe in that approach, I have carefully listed the most common items you might have in your fridge or in your pantry. For each of them I have not only listed their calorie count, but also the quantity of Proteins, Fat, Carbs and Fibers they contain.

Macro Tracking

In macro tracking strategy (or tracking your daily macronutrient intake), you focus on calories from protein, carbohydrates, and fat throughout your day. If you stay within your limit of those three macronutrients, you will hit your calorie goal as well.

Both basic calorie intake tracking and tracking your macro intake have you keeping track of a few variables (your calorie intake from different sources). While basic calorie intake tracking has you watching and tracking your calorie intake regardless of source, tracking your macro intake focuses on protein, carbohydrates, and fat intake; that is the only real difference between the two.

Protein Tracking

This strategy is where we start to get specialized with how we view our calorie intake from day to day.

Protein tracking focuses on just that: Protein. This doesn't mean you

want all of your calories to come from just protein (aside from that being damn near impossible, it is also incredibly unhealthy), but rather has you focus on hitting a daily protein goal then lets you fill in the rest of your daily calorie intake.

This strategy is primarily used for muscle gain ("glamour" muscles or otherwise), but also helps you reach and maintain your target weight. To use this strategy, you simply set a calorie goal but set the emphasis on meeting a protein-calorie goal within that.

Protein becomes your priority and then carbohydrates and fats fill in the rest of your daily calorie intake without worrying too much about how much of either goes into your body (as long as they stay within your limit).

Portion Control and Tracking

Rather than counting individual calories throughout a normal day, the portion control strategy has you tracking the daily portions of protein, carbohydrates, and fat you intake throughout a given day. This means that rather than set a goal for 20 calories from protein a day, you want to eat two servings of protein a day.

It should be noted that this strategy might take a bit of practice and alteration to make it fit your personal style and goals. A common suggestion is to learn how many calories of protein, carbohydrates, and fats come in a serving and use those numbers to determine your daily portion intake goals.

Yes, using this strategy can be similar to counting calories because, basically, you are counting calories in another way (converting calories to portions and tracking portion intake). However, once you get the hang of counting portions rather than calories directly, and can do so without thinking about it, you may find it a lot easier and, in some cases, a lot more stress free.

Single Meal Tracking and Moderate Fasting

Single meal tracking revolves around the idea that you enjoy a single large meal in a day (usually breakfast or the first meal you eat) and enjoy smaller meals throughout, to best keep your weight down. If this sounds familiar, it should, because it's very closely related to the myths about eating several small meals or not eating large meals.

What single meal tracking ideally does is allow for a metabolic kick in the morning that you ride out for a good portion of the day while you keep your metabolism relatively high (while keeping yourself from getting too hungry); by eating small snacks throughout the rest of the morning and afternoon into the evening. By doing this, you allow your body to burn off the energy it gained from that large breakfast, then continue to burn off energy and fat after that. The snacks, while providing the calories (and energy) you need, allow your body to maintain that higher metabolic rate while keeping your calorie count lower, which in turn continues to burn excess fat from your body.

Moderate fasting means that you can plan specific days to involve a large meal early on, then eat next to nothing for another meal. This portion of the strategy is very similar to the first part about tracking a single large meal. The only real difference is the emphasis on calorie intake throughout the day.

While single meal tracking suggests you eat a large meal early on, moderate fasting means that you may eat a decently sized breakfast, a very small lunch, and nothing for dinner.

CHAPTER 10:

Supplementation

Many of those who are doing an intermittent fast for either weight loss or health reasons wonder whether it is a good idea for them to take a dietary supplement during that time. The worries for this include whether they actually need the nutrition that can come from these supplements and whether this supplement will break their fast and ruin all their efforts.

Are supplements needed?

Taking a supplement is not always a requirement, though. You can quickly go on an intermittent fast without having to worry about taking these supplements, as long as you pick out a meal plan or a diet that will provide you with these nutrients. But since getting these nutrients can be difficult for those who are starting on an intermittent fast for the first time, or because you want to make sure that you can get the full benefits of a fast, you may want to get at least some supplements to help start your fast.

There are times when taking a supplement, such as during the beginning of the fast as you adjust, can be a good idea to help you out.

One of the benefits that you get with fasting is that while you are doing it, this process is going to put your body in a state that is known as autophagy. This is where the body is cleaning itself out. Most people never give their bodies enough of a break to experience this natural cleansing of the body.

Now, for the most part, you should avoid taking any supplement when you are in the fasting state to allow the body to go through this cleansing process that you want. But there are some types of supplements that you can take that will help enhance and sometimes speed up this process of autophagy. For example, resveratrol is a supplement that can do this. If you choose to take this supplement, it helps to take it at the beginning of the fast and then again the next morning.

What type of supplements?

In addition to considering some supplements to enhance the results that you get during the fast, there are also some supplements that you can consider taking when you enter your eating window. These should not be taken during your fasting period because they effectively end the fast, but they can help you give your body the right nutrients when you enter your eating window. Proteins, in the form of whey, and branched chain amino acids are excellent options and can immediately tell the body that it is time to end the fast.

There are essential nutrients that you can work with that will either enhance the fasting state or will help keep your body staying healthy while you are fasting. There is a wide variety of different supplements though, and most people don't want to go through and keep all these on hand.

If you choose to start on a multivitamin, make sure that you get one that is high quality and one that has, at a minimum, the nutrients that are listed above. Take it when you break your fast, right at breakfast that day, to get them absorbed into the body as soon as possible.

While you are doing intermittent fasting, your body breaks down all the dead cells and other waste materials that are already in your body. This process creates some energy, and it even gives you most of the macronutrients that you may require for short-term survival.

When you fast for more extended periods, your body triggers autophagy and metabolic pathways that help your body to release micronutrients from mineral stores. Before that, you will be getting enough nutrients from food, given that you are eating non-processed foods. Therefore, you do not need to take lots of nutrients if you are eating a wide range of foods. But there are some supplements you can choose if you feel that you are deficient in some minerals and nutrients.

Some other supplements that you can take that will help you provide the body with the right amount of nutrition and should be taken when you are in your eating window include:

Resveratrol (Essential)

This is a good option that you can take during your fasted state, usually right at the beginning and then again halfway through.

Magnesium (Essential)

Magnesium is a body mineral that regulates several vital body functions. Magnesium helps to regulate nerve and blood pressure and is easily and swiftly depleted in the period of fasting. Low magnesium is what can cause the feeling of brain fogginess or muscle cramps during a fasting period. You can begin your fasted state with a full dose of this. Try to take in this supplement as close to your bedtime as possible to get the best effects.

Omega-3 fatty acids (Essential)

You can quickly get enough of these from the fish that you should be eating. But if you are taking a supplement, take it at the start of your eating window.

Vitamin K (Essential)

You can take this one at the beginning of your eating window. This is an important one to get in because it helps you process calcium in the body.

IP6 (Essential)

You want to take this one at the end of your eating window, right when you are entering a fast. Or you can take it when you are getting ready for bed, and your stomach is empty.

Glucosamine (Not Essential)

You can take this towards the end of your eating window.

Astaxanthin (Not Essential)

This should be taken along with your first meal after you break a fast.

Nicotinamide (Not Essential)

You can take this supplement when you are in the middle of your fast. This supplement is going to help you enhance the effects of the fast.

Hydroxycitrate (Not Essential)

You can also take this one during the middle of your fasting time to help you get more out of the impact.

Curcumin (Not Essential)

This is one that you can take when you are ready to break a fast. Take it with that first meal when it is time to break the fast.

Sodium and Potassium (Essential)

Levels of ketones in the bloodstream rise during your periods of fasting, which cause your body to signal a flushing response. This quickly depletes the stores of potassium and sodium. It can cause fatigue, low energy, and the feeling of being lightheaded. These minerals are essential for ketogenesis, and without them, the body really must work and struggle to access the stores of fat.

B-Complex Vitamins (Essential)

B-complex vitamin, which includes riboflavin, niacin, thiamine, and biotin are vitamins that aid the body in absorbing nutrients. B-complex vitamins do not get flushed out of the body in the same way sodium, potassium, and magnesium does during the state of ketosis. However, there are a large number of women who are chronically low or have B-complex vitamin deficiencies.

Vitamin D (Essential)

Vitamin D is a prevalent deficiency amongst both men and women. Vitamin D is rather difficult to obtain through food intake and is acquired naturally through sunlight. Vitamin D is vital to both immune health and bone density. Vitamin D helps the use of nutrients that are critical to body functions and help allow the nutrients to function, magnesium being one of them.

Chromium (Not Essential)

Chromium is not as common in your everyday multivitamin, but there has been some research that shows it can be a culprit that mitigates hunger. This can be problematic as it may force you to end your fast earlier than planned or expected due to the hunger pangs.

Beta-Hydroxybutyrate or BHB (Not Essential)

Many women who intermittently fast also take a BHB supplement as well; these are also known as exogenous ketones. This means ketones that are not produced by the body. One of the three ketone bodies is BHB. Ketone bodies are naturally produced by the liver when you are in a state of ketosis. If broken down to the cellular level, the human body needs BHB to access and adequately use the fat stores for energy. Using a BHB supplement during a fast helps to ensure that the body will have the necessary levels of BHB in the bloodstream. Having the proper levels of BHB in the bloodstream will help to facilitate the metabolizing of fat into energy.

CHAPTER 11:

The Biggest Mistakes To Avoid

When asked about their nutrition, the answer always reveals the problem. They are still eating processed foods (chips, candy, cake, crackers, etc.) and drinking sweetened beverages (sweet teas and soda). You cannot fast, exercise hard, eat junk food, and still expect that you will lose fat and tone that butt. You must decide to throw away all the unhealthy stuff and go for whole and unprocessed foods.

Eating too much in the Feeding Period

Eating too much food after a fast period is a common mistake. The stomach has a certain amount of dispensability. While in a fast, it contracts and adapts to handling less. When you are eating a lot, it develops and gets used to accommodating more significant amounts of food. When you are preparing to break your fast, you naturally want to eat heavy foods that are very dense but you should control it by eating less food during this period until the body gets used to food.

Not Drinking Enough Water

Another common mistake is not keeping yourself hydrated enough. Many times, when you feel like you may be hungry, it may be your body telling you to hydrate it. The body also demands more salt on an intermittent fasting diet. Be sure to get enough water and salt as these are essential to getting good, healthy results. Studies state that you should drink 8-ounce glasses of water daily. Drinking enough water and staying well hydrated also helps to prevent and get over the flu, if you are also following the ketogenic diet. Hydration is key to any change in diet and will nearly always improve your results.

Quitting before you give intermittent fasting a fighting chance

It's a lifestyle! Yes - it's a challenging transition, but the potential rewards are AMAZING! I've read many an account of people who have fasted for two and a half hours and called it quits. For Pete's sake, everyone can fast for at least 6 hours right out of the box. How do I know that? Because even the worst sleeper (have I mentioned that intermittent fasting could improve your sleep?) has had a "restful" 6 hours of sleep every once in a while.

I'm going to ask you to please give intermittent fasting at least 30 days – one month to try it out and experience the changes it makes. And please don't limit yourself only to pounds lost.

Going the whole Hog on your first fast

There is no humiliation in easing into intermittent fasting. Take advantage of the many different intermittent fasting plans in existence and "date" a couple of them before making a big commitment. You may find that several ideas resonate more than others, and want to mix and match plans or create your hybrid. Just remember the golden rules: No more than two 24-hour period fasts per week, and no two 24-hour fasts on consecutive days. For time restrictive plans, don't go more than 16 hours each day without feeding for the balance of the 24 hours.

Alternatively, design your gradual immersion schedule to acclimate yourself to intermittent fasting gracefully. You could accomplish this either by gradually extending the periods you fast or by decreasing progressively the hours you feed.

You sit around and wait for the result

Especially when you first start intermittently fasting, it's highly advisable to keep your mind and body doing something so you don't sit around obsessing on the fact that you can't eat. Don't clear your schedule for your first fast. Live your life and let it fill you instead of food. Try and schedule activities that aren't about food in any way. Avoid break rooms and snack cabinets at the office. Take a miss on the third birthday party cake-fest this week! Give yourself a break and take a nice long walk. Watch your favorite comfort show on Netflix or permit yourself to take a well-deserved afternoon nap. You will be amazed, and perhaps a bit startled by how much food there is in western culture; how we idolize it, covet it and include it every time we gather to mark an important event; be it a joyous wedding or a somber funeral. It will give you pause – take that pause to reflect and decide how much you want food in your life.

Going overboard with the "stimulants"

So, caffeine in the form of coffee and tea is allowed when you intermittently fast, and that's a good thing. Remember the whole balance thing, so your pleasant morning coffee "euphoria" doesn't turn into a raging case of café nervosa! Too much caffeine will wreak havoc with your stomach and nervous system. Drink coffee and tea mindfully, always keeping your tolerance levels in mind.

Fasting for many days per week

Sometimes if your goal for adopting intermittent fasting is to lose weight, then it's possible to go out of your way to ensure that you lose it fast. Such an ambition can drive one into engaging in practices that are likely to cause more problems. Fasting can be done at least for 2 – 4 days and anything more than that can be quite exhausting. Fasting for many days within a week can also impact on your metabolism, body performance, and appetite. Your body can also start defending itself against the perceived starvation and that might lead to the release of some hunger hormones which has the potential of causing hormonal imbalance, especially in women.

It's vital that one makes use of the fasting window when participating in intermittent fasting. When the window period is too large, then that can also trigger high hunger levels, which then results in uncontrolled eating and even bingeing. The fasting protocol that one gets to choose, therefore plays such an integral part in helping one to stay focused on the fasting process in a way that enables them to realize their goals.

Intense training while fasting

Another common mistake that most people make during intermittent fasting is engaging in intense training as they also fast. As much as some people may not have any problems with intense training and workout during fasting, there are those who are likely to suffer very negative consequences. Fasting is generally fierce for the body and taking time to rest or even engage in some light exercises such as yoga, can be appropriate. However, if it's intense such as the lifting of weights, then one should choose shorter fasting periods so that the body gets replenished with carbohydrates after engaging in such intense training.

Instead of engaging in intense work out during the fasting period, one can consider participating in restorative workouts like taking a walk or even yoga as we have shared. Such mild exercises are also great at preventing feelings of dizziness, weakness, and fatigue. Another important thing that one should look into during the fasting period is to ensure they get enough sleep. Sufficient sleep is vital as it enables the body to repair itself while you also maintain healthy digestion, hormonal balance, and detoxification, amongst other things. You should at least aim to sleep for about 7 – 9 hours to prevent low energy, moodiness, and cravings.

Sufficient sleep is quite essential since growth hormones usually get released during the first hours of sleep. If you spend your time on gadgets and other distracting things, then you are more likely to feel fatigued the following day and may lack the required strength and focus on going through the fasting time effectively.

Ignoring body temperature changes when fasting

Some people experience an internal temperature drop when fasting. This is a stress response. Dress warmly and don't push yourself in any way that would add additional stressors to your day.

In terms of intermittent fasting, MORE does not equal BETTER: There is an excellent, scientific reason why you shouldn't fast more than two full days a week. Simply put, most benefits of intermittent fasting decline at the whole day mark. If you find yourself stretching out your fasting periods past the recommended times, you need to rethink things. This would be a good place to consider the difference between fasting and starvation.

In terms of intermittent feeding, LESS does not equal MORE: Be very careful not to start cutting down on your food intake to see if you can lose more weight faster. Intermittent fasting is about moderation and balance between fasting and feeding. Don't tip this beautiful balance by cheating yourself out of the food you need to stay healthy. If you feel like this might be happening, seek medical help immediately!

Stalking the clock

Most newbies will develop an obsession with the clock when fasting. They will count down the hours, minutes, and seconds until they can rush to the kitchen and start bingeing. On the other end are people who are afraid of breaking the "rules," so they make sure that they fast until the last second of the fasting window is over. Intermittent fasting is not that hard or strict. You cannot spend the day worrying and wondering about the timeframes and schedules. If your entire life starts and ends with your next meal, you will drive yourself mad. Just relax and enjoy the ride.

If you fall into this category, try and reinforce the flexibility of fasting by deregulating the exact times you eat during your feeding window. Experiment with snacking. Vary your mealtimes and make allowances for social interaction and special events. Be mindful about developing rigidity around eating.

Not Having Enough Support

Often with any diet, this is the most significant cause of failure. Support for a life change is absolutely a necessity. Without having a support system to lean on, ask questions, and discuss ideas with, most people are unsuccessful. If you are struggling and frustrated, be sure to find someone who is also going through the changes and adjustments that come with changing your habits to an intermittent fasting lifestyle. There are many online support groups with excellent support systems and knowledge to share. Changing your life is hard as it is, and it is nearly impossible to do alone.

Not Keeping Yourself Busy

You cannot spend the day fasting and sitting around doing nothing. Staying idle is the worst thing you can do because you will start thinking about food. Get up and do something to keep active, as long as it keeps you away from food.

Setting Goals Too High

 If you are a newbie to intermittent fasting, make sure that you don't start with only one meal a day. You may think that going in hard from the start will help you torch all that fat, but it doesn't work that way. You cannot go from eating four to six meals a day to surviving on a single meal.

You Fear Going Hungry

Learn to recognize and come to terms with casual hunger. Know, with the growing assurance that comes with acclimating yourself to intermittent fasting, that occasional hunger is a passing thing. You know to understand that short term fasting doesn't cause the body to "devour its own" muscle tissue or create any other bodily harm. Don't let your mind play games with your intentions.

It's perfectly normal to feel hungry, but you will not die just because you go for a couple of hours without food. Most people have this irrational and morbid fear of depriving themselves of food, believing that all their muscles will be gobbled up. This fear can tempt you to cheat during your fasting window. Do not be afraid of a bit of hunger.

CHAPTER 12:

Differences Between Men And Women Intermittent Fasting

While intermittent fasting is flexible, versatile, and adaptable to many different lifestyles, it is still the case that many women should probably not attempt IF, for the sake of their overall health. Women practice intermittent fasting to lose weight and men practice intermittent fasting to build muscle.

Women and Intermittent Fasting

Intermittent fasting is a great plan that helps women to reduce their calories and increase their metabolism all in one. There are many ways to do an intermittent fast, which makes it easy for almost everyone to go on one of these fasts. While many women have gone on an intermittent fast and believe that it is one of the best things that they have ever done, there are other women who find that there were severe problems with fasting including loss of menstrual periods, metabolic disruption, binge eating, and even early onset menopause. And these could happen to women who are as young as their mid-20s.

So, is it safe for women to go on an intermittent fast? The answer is; it depends. Many women are going to respond to intermittent fasting differently than men, and it often depends on how hard they go into the active fast and which type of fasting program they decide to go on. If you plan to start with an intermittent fast as a woman, it is essential that you understand how this eating plan can affect you and what precautions you should take to do a fast safely.

The female hormones and fasting

Many people think that intermittent fasting is not a big deal and that experimenting with it a bit isn't such a big deal. But for some women, small decisions can have a significant impact on them. The hormones that can regulate some critical functions in women, such as ovulation, are going to be incredibly sensitive to the amount of energy that you take in.

In both genders, the hypothalamic-pituitary gonadal axis, which is the cooperative functioning of three endocrine glands, can act similar to how you would imagine an air traffic controller. First, your hypothalamus is going to release a hormone that is known as GnRH. This is then going to tell your pituitary gland to release the LH hormone and the FHS hormone.

These two hormones are going to act on the gonads of the individual, which would be either the ovaries or the testes. In women, this means that these hormones are going to trigger the production of progesterone and estrogen, both of which are needed to help release a mature egg and to help support a pregnancy. For men, these hormones are going to trigger the production of testosterone and sperm production.

Because of this chain of reaction that occur at a specific time to make a regular cycle in women, the GnRH pulses need to be timed or they can get everything off. But these pulses are going to be sensitive to environmental factors, and if you are not careful, they are going to be thrown off with fasting. Even some short term fasting, such as three days, can alter these pulses in some women.

This is not entirely clear yet. This kisspeptin is going to stimulate the production of GnRH in both sexes, and it can be susceptible to ghrelin, insulin, and leptin, the hormones that will regulate and react to satiety and hunger.

What is interesting is that females often produce more of this kisspeptin than males. The more kisspeptin neurons that are in the body, the higher sensitivity there is to changes in energy balance. This could be a big reason why females are going to have more trouble with fasting.

For many women, the solution is to cut down on how long your fasting window is. Many men can do the Warrior diet or do alternate day fasting, but this may be a bit intense for most women, especially when they first get started on fasting. You may want to consider working with either a 5:2 diet or do the 16/8 diet. These are less extreme when you first get started so your body can get used to the idea, without a big shock to the system. If you respond well to those and want to move over to alternate day fasting or another option over time, then you can consider it when you know how your body will react.

You can see better results when you spend more time fasting daily.

There is no specific chart – you can fast as frequently as you prefer. The more you fast, the more effective the result.

When you follow Intermittent fasting, you gain more health benefits apart from weight loss. How does your body lose weight when you fast? Your body uses the stored body fat for energy. This results in burning all the unwanted calories. When you burn calories in this way, you lose weight and also burn the excess fat. This will help you get a lean physique, and you will also feel healthy and energetic, as the body uses the excess body fat for energy. This is because it doesn't get power from the food intake since your food intake is restricted.

Intermittent fasting helps your body to optimize the release of the major fat burning hormones – especially insulin and HGH (Human Growth Hormone) – the two most important ones. Human Growth Hormone is responsible for switching on your body's fat burning system. Your body starts to burn all the excess fat to give you the energy to carry on with your regular work (routine).

Intermittent fasting also has a significant influence on the other important hormone – insulin. It helps to keep the insulin levels steady and low, which is key to losing excess weight or avoiding extra fat from becoming accumulated in the body. Foods rich in processed carbohydrates and pure sugar accumulate more body fat. It is therefore advisable to avoid these foods as it causes the insulin levels to skyrocket and then crash whenever you eat them. This will result in excess fat accumulation in your body instead of burning it as energy.

When your insulin levels go up, you end up with health issues like obesity, Type II diabetes, and various other chronic health conditions. Intermittent fasting is the solution to all these problems. Clinical studies have proven that 15 days of consistent intermittent fasting helps to balance insulin levels.

Women who should avoid intermittent fasting

Pregnant Women - This is because pregnant women have a higher demand for more energy and nutrients that come from what they eat and drink. But really, some women should not even try experimenting with intermittent fasting at all. If you do not feast or fast correctly, you risk becoming infertile or having early onset menopause: also if you are in your twenties. Fasting and feasting could lead to unhealthy eating patterns which will cause additional problems.

Although intermittent fasting can give you increased energy, better metabolism, and stronger cellular protection, the risks outweigh the benefits for pregnant IF candidates. Since the female body is made to bear children, the effects of intermittent fasting are already debated in their relation to female health, but when it comes to pregnant and soon-to-be mothers, the answer to the question is a definite "No." Pregnant women should not be intermittent fasting.

For the expecting mother, long periods between meals are not necessarily such a good thing. The pregnant woman will need to be eating whenever she's hungry to gain the weight and nutrients her future child will need to survive. Furthermore, she will need to combat the morning sickness and nausea that go along with pregnancy, and if she's concerned about her timing with the intermittent fast, she might put herself in a detrimental situation for her overall health by mistake.

If you're recently pregnant but had used intermittent fasting previously with great success, you can shift back to focusing on what you eat rather than when you eat. Just as it is for the standard person moving from healthy eating to intermittent fasting and going from what's eaten to when it's eaten, when you switch from IF to pregnancy, you'll shift eating habits once again. This time, however, you'll try to make sure you're eating the best foods whenever possible; not just in your okayed eating windows.

If you're having trouble stopping your intermittent fast while you've just become pregnant, you might want to reconsider the reasons behind your IF in the first place. Is it really for your health, or does it support your controlling tendency to limit your weight? Try to make sure that when you're pregnant, you're looking for what supports your health, rather than your mental image of what you should look like and what you think you should weigh.

Underweight women - For women who are already skinny, intermittent fasting might not be the best thing for your health. Admittedly, there are unintentionally thin women who don't have the time they'd like to have for eating or who don't have the energy they'd like to have for cooking, but there are also intentionally underweight women who are looking for an additional method to use to keep off that "excess" weight for good.

If you're incredibly underweight already (even if you don't feel like it!), steer clear of intermittent fasting. If you're only five to ten pounds underweight and you're seeking spiritual enlightenment, lessened brain fog, or a jolt to your digestive system, IF may work just fine for you without being problematic.

Women with Eating Disorder - For the individual with an eating disorder, no matter what variety, intermittent fasting may seem to be helpful, because it will only function as a trigger for that person's disease. No matter who you are, if you approach intermittent fasting for healing or weight loss, you're probably doing so because you want to switch from stuffing yourself of emptiness to healing yourself with goodness. Your focus, in other words, likely falls on growth (not physically but emotionally, spiritually, mentally, and regarding health capacity) rather than withering.

Question their inspirations and drives; demand they are honest with you. The likelihood is more significant than not that this person is using intermittent fasting as a way to lose weight; they can't afford to lose rather than to get healthier in general. If you're able to discern it at all, the individual's reason for starting IF is the best way to ascertain their true intentions. It can be hard to tell who has an eating disorder and who doesn't, but the way people talk about food, body image, fasting, and dieting can reveal more than you could ever anticipate. And once you can tell who has an eating disorder, help them stay clear from IF because it can exacerbate their circumstances despite their (and your) best intentions.

Diabetic women - If you're already on insulin, as a diabetic most likely, you're already working to keep your levels of blood sugar at balance. If you add into the mix IF work to increase or decrease insulin resistance (to help with weight loss), you'll put yourself in a hazardous spot. People with diabetes should not skip doses of insulin to lose weight by lowering blood sugar. This would be disastrous for someone who has diabetes because they'd surely lose the weight, but they'd feel drained to a devastating degree because humans do need this sugar or glucose in our blood to derive energy.

So, if you have diabetes, stay away from intermittent fasting. As with the pregnant candidate, you could try to switch the foods you're eating instead of when you're eating. By adding the right, healthful foods into your diet, you might find that the weight that sticks to you so stubbornly can be depleted with your condition being made none the worse. However, be careful if you have diabetes when it comes to fasting disguised as dieting. If you feel inclined to try a juice or liquid diet, second guess those inclinations, for it's very likely that this type of food would cause extra stress to your system, what with the high glycemic and fiber-free contents of some juices.

If you have diabetes and feel inclined to make your life healthier, don't limit when you eat and don't just drink liquids. Rather than restricting whatsoever, try to incorporate healthier, more whole foods that are oriented towards healing innately and then maybe add exercise into the mix when you're ready for it.

Other women who should not consider intermittent fasting are:

Those who are chronically stressed or do not handle physical or mental stress well - people who experience constant chronic stress should not limit their diet or meals because they may need more nourishment.

Women who suffer from insomnia or unusual sleeping habits – Just like individuals with chronic stress, and if you have trouble sleeping, then you need to be nurturing your body not adding more stress to it.

If you are new to exercising and dieting and this is the first time you are trying a new lifestyle.

Intermittent Fasting for men

Intermittent fasting has shown to be just as useful as a regular calorie-restrictive diet in many ways. However, men who choose the intermittent fasting route have been seen to preserve muscle mass while losing fat, while groups following a calorie-restricted diet for the same period lost both fat and muscle mass. There are a few ways to optimize muscle gain while on an intermittent fasting diet. It is essential to remember to consult a doctor before implementing any fasting regimens into your daily routine, especially when the goal results involve drastic weight loss or muscle growth. The most important key is to ensure that you are eating enough calories during your feeding hours to compensate for calories lost during workouts.

The primary difference between trying to lose weight while fasting and trying to gain muscle while fasting is the way you exercise and the food you cat. Intermittent fasting is a beneficial tool when trying to gain muscle because you can lose fat and build muscle at the same time. The fasting is taking care of the fat loss, so you do not have to worry as much about burning fat in your diet and workouts. This changes the way you approach training. Your focus isn't on toning up to look better, it's on pushing your limits and getting stronger.

If you are doing bicep curls and 45 pounds is the maximum amount that you can successfully curl only once, then you need to be using at least 18 pounds for each set of reps to be building muscle. 60 percent of a single rep max is generally an amount that you can lift between 15 and 20 times in one set. This is not a particularly heavyweight, but as a beginner, it will help you build muscle.

As your body adjusts to lifting weights, consistently it becomes more difficult to build muscle. Over time, you will need to increase the percentage to at least 80 percent of your max to still be getting stronger and growing muscle. This is going to be an amount that you can't lift as many times. Rather than being able to do 15 to 20 reps in one set, you are not likely to be able to surpass 8 or 9 reps before you can't do anymore. So, the amount of weight you lift will affect muscle growth.

Many people encourage slow, deliberate reps when trying to get stronger. This may help maintain proper form, but it is not as effective in building functional strength or optimal muscle growth. Maintain controlled movements, but lift the weight faster and lower it slowly. Boosting faster yields more optimal muscle growth results because it uses more muscle fibers. This increases the amount of damage to the cells in the muscles, which in turn increases the number of new, healthy cells that are added to repair them. So, lift heavier weights and lift them faster, but always maintain proper form.

If you reach a point in your sets where you cannot complete the reps without cheating on your form, stop. Reduce the weight if you'd like to finish out the game, but do not continue if you can't do it properly. Not using proper form can cause stress and injury to the muscles. When you are lifting heavy, you are working your most muscular tissues. When these stop doing their part, weaker muscle fibers start to bear a weight they are not cut out for. Damaging the muscles is part of building them, but injuring them is not a factor we want to add to the equation.

Muscles grow when you feed them. When trying to add muscle while fasting, you will need to increase the number of calories consumed during the feeding hours. On days involving exercise, make sure the body is fed a surplus of calories so it can have the necessary fuel to perform protein biosynthesis. During training, muscle fibers are damaged. The body is always clearing out old, damaged cells and adding newer, healthier ones, so these damaged muscle cells get replaced with new ones. The body also has a nifty skill called adaptability. It wants to become better suited to dealing with whatever stimulus caused the damage to muscle fibers, so when the muscle fibers are repaired, the body adds extra cells. This causes the muscles to get bigger. This is why bodybuilding athletes consume so much protein. The goal is to ensure that the body synthesizes more protein than is broken down. If more protein is destroyed than is being made, you will begin to lose muscle mass.

When you are fasting and trying to build muscle, you do not want a large calorie deficit. Instead, to gain muscle mass, you need to have a caloric surplus. This means that you'll need to increase the number of calories you eat during your feeding window, but that does not mean you should start stuffing your face with junk food to meet the necessary surplus.

By adopting a weight training routine combined with your elevated hormones you will be able to add lean muscle faster than you thought was possible. Not to mention that the act of lifting weights also increases testosterone and growth hormone production, so your body will be getting a double dose of hormone production.

Weight training is also highly metabolic so you will shred the fat from your body because more muscle = less fat.

I highly suggest you start exercising and if you don't have a gym that's fine – bodyweight exercises such as push-ups, air squats, lunges **etc.** will all aid you in your journey.

CHAPTER 13:

Signs That You Have To Stop Fasting

As with anything in life, intermittent fasting, though severely beneficial to your health, also has its share of drawbacks. As such, it may not be as helpful to certain people.

There are times when you will want to consider stopping an intermittent fast. Even if you follow some of the advice that we give in this book, you may want to stop intermittent fasting if it is not working for you. Most people are going to do well with an intermittent fast if they are careful and don't prolong them for too long. But others are more sensitive to the changes in their hormones, and intermittent fasting can make this worse. Here are a few precautions to keep in mind when considering intermittent fasting.

- You feel cold all the time.

- You can notice if your digestion is slowing down.

- Your interest in romance fizzles, and you don't appreciate it at all.

- Your heart starts to feel rapid and pitter patter in a strange way.

- You see a lot of mood swings suddenly.

- You notice that your tolerance for any stress has decreased.

- When you get an injury, you are slow to heal, or you get a bug every time it comes around.

- When you finish with a workout, you aren't recovering as well as you should.

- You start to develop a lot of acne or dry skin.

- Your hair starts to fall out.

- You aren't able to fall asleep very well, and you have trouble staying asleep.

- Your menstrual cycle becomes irregular, or you find that it stops completely.

Don'ts of Intermittent Fasting

Avoid Excessive Eating

A night before your fast, concentrate on healthy and lean protein, lots of vegetables and fat. We recommend starchy foods like sweet potato and legumes. You can also get natural sugar via fruits, which could help relax your hormones. Foods, low on the glycemic index like berry, is a good idea.

Your aim should be a nutritious food that your body will slowly burn and absorb the nutrient gradually. This will carry you through your fasting period rather than feasting on heavy meals.

Don't try to be a perfectionist

So, what would you do if you polished off a bag of Oreos? Perfectionist thinking gets in the way of success more than any other factor. If a 200-calorie indulgence is just that, "an indulgence" and nothing more, then it's okay. However, if you perceive it as a failure and a reason to give up, it can quickly turn into a 1000-calorie indulgence. Don't try to be a perfectionist when you start to diet. As mentioned in the previous tip, setbacks are expected and you should deal with them in a positive way.

Don't be too hard on yourself

When you are first starting out, it is important to not only understand that the transitional period can be rough for some people but also to understand what that means for you. While it is certainly important to hold yourself accountable in order to ensure that you don't make poor choices in the long run, when you are first starting out, there is no reason to be ashamed if you only make it 13 hours instead of 14. The transition period is going to be difficult enough with the very real physical issues you will be dealing with, you don't need to add additional mental stress to the mix as well.

Do Not Expect to See Miracles!

This is a mistake that every beginner makes when he or she starts any fast. You will want to see results in a week or two. But what they forget is that a fast is not the only thing that will help. You need to understand the fact that there are many other factors that will affect the way you lose weight, or even the amount of weight you will lose. You have to look at intermittent fasting, along with other healthy habits, like exercise and sleep, which will ensure that you lose weight consistently.

Don't Push Too Hard on Fasting Days

If you choose to work out on the days that you fast, it will be vital that you listen to what your body is saying to you. Exercising can be difficult while fasting as you tend to get feelings of light headedness, and a lack of stamina to drive performance. If you find that you begin to experience this, ensure that you are fully hydrated and that while in your 'feeding windows' you are hitting the correct number of calories that you should be for your specific body mass index. If you are, evaluate what it is that you are eating to hit this caloric mark. You want to ensure that most of your calories are coming from healthy fats, and protein.

Avoid Being a Hero

There can be side effects of fasting. As we have said several times, listen to your body. You are not trying to impress anyone by doing one meal a day fast, nor are you in competition with anyone. If you start experiencing dizziness, heart palpitations, and weakness, you need to take a step back. If you are too weak to go about your daily tasks, it is not a crime to stop the fast.

Avoid Stress

Be sure to take time to relax. Take time to engage in stress-busting activities for your fast if you want satisfactory results. Stress-busting activities like deep breathing, yoga, and meditation are all a good idea, whether fasting or not. You can also go for a walk, as a walk to the beach or park can have a calming effect on your nerves.

CHAPTER 14:

How To Cheat During Intermittent Fasting

Intermittent fasting intended to bring about weight loss or whatever else may be its goal, always takes some time before the dieter realizes the results and stops. In the course of this, it is necessary to do some cheating; implying that it may be planned prior to the fasting begins to have a specific time to act contrary to the standards of this-this fasting. For example, to enjoy your special meal which is not on the fasting diet plan, to enjoy meals with friends or family which occasionally violate the set fasting requirements but are necessary for social and other personal reasons.

There will be cheat days when you can indulge in something decadent, but don't make that part of your intermittent fasting lifestyle. So, you've been intermittently fasting religiously. You've got the timing down to the second, and you never cheat…during the fast. But when it's feeding time, all bets are off, and any indulgence is fair game.

If you have heard of people cheating during fasting or when following a diet program, it is not so much as a result of hunger as it is a result of cravings. Many people could easily overcome desire but seem unable to resist cravings. This is both a biological and psychological effect of abstaining from food.

Biologically, your body's search for glucose is heightened in the early days of keeping away from food. When you fast, there is no supply of glucose to the body through your regular and timely meals and snacks. This glucose hunt is what makes you begin to crave foods that have high sugar content or are high in other carbohydrates.

An arrangement to this effect should be made so that some specific time is set aside, for instance, one day a week so that it caters for this arrangement. After all, this single occasion or very few of them a week will not prevent your intermittent fasting goal. Cheat time is ideal because:

• It helps you to satisfy your taste buds in case you crave certain food items,

• It enables the dieter to go on for a longer time because they don't miss anything

• It keeps your social life relatively active

• It activates metabolism and leptin, which are slowed down during the daily fasting routine.

It should be noted that cheat days/meals do not promote weight gain because they are just an occasional arrangement.

CHAPTER 15:

Organic Or Non-Organic Food- What Should You Eat

When you hear organic, you surely know – minus synthetic fertilizers. You also appreciate it is minus pesticides. Again correct. Now, those are the two factors that distinguish organic foods from non-organic ones. But you realize that the farmer would need to disclose those facts to you otherwise you would not know how the food was grown. Still, the farmer might be gracious enough to disclose to a store owner the fact that the food is not organic, but the trader might decide to veil that fact behind some jargon.

Organic foods contain organic and not artificial materials. The set standards for these foods vary from one country to another but they must all follow whatever regulations are set.

Organic foods aren't strictly fruits and vegetables as many may tend to believe.

So, are there any physical signs that can tell you, as a consumer, that certain food is likely to be organic or not? Yes, luckily, there are. Like the innocent, genuine village folk, organic food may not have much cosmetic appeal, but it distinctly tastes great. A good example are the organic carrots that have a rugged look that could sometimes make you frown, but which are sweet in an irresistible way.

And on that note, you might wonder, why not try and change that rather rough look of many organic foods? Well, you do not want to go that way because it would be copying the growers of foods of that are not organic; those who use chemical material to wax their products smooth.

Here are attractive features of organic food:

It is healthy. By eating organic, you drastically lower the chance of disease that is triggered by use of chemicals and other synthetic products on crops and animals. Such diseases include the dreaded cancer.

Higher in nutrition. What does that mean, considering that there is no mention of the main nutrients – protein, carbohydrates and fats?

It is not genetically modified. Antioxidants effectively clean your body cells, thus making your body not susceptible to disease. Just like a dirty floor draws pests, when your body is full of bad elements, otherwise referred to as free radicals, it is great ground for disease causing organisms. And those free radicals are the ones that get cleared by the antioxidants. So we are talking of organic foods helping to keep your hospital bills in check; and, of course, you being able to lead a healthy life.

Why You Need to Eat Organic Foods

As long as you realize that inorganic foods are an easy gateway to disease, you will want to go for organic. There are actually direct and indirect advantages of pursuing organic foods. If many of you eat organic, more and more farmers will be motivated to produce food organically. You will thereby enjoy:

A cleaner environment. This is because organic farming uses organic pest control substances as opposed to artificial insecticides. As a result, you have clean water sources and green fodder for your animals. This, you need to appreciate, is not a scholarly report that needs detailed analysis. Right from where you are, if you and your immediate neighbors are into organic farming, you will rarely find your families needing medical attention.

Reduced pollution. Having organic farming is a great way to keep away diseases that come about from environmental pollution. You do not breathe dangerous gases from artificial pesticides and herbicides. That, obviously, implies a healthier and more productive life for you and your family.

Water and soil conservation. When you eat organic and farmers stick to organic farming, what happens to the soil texture is very positive because there are no chemicals that would destroy it. On the other hand, manure that is used in place of synthetic fertilizers help to enrich the soil organically, leaving it strong in nutrients and in texture. As a result, the soil retains water longer, and food supply becomes more reliable than otherwise.

Improving financial position. Did you know that every time you save on cost, it is like you are actually earning more income? Think of the amount of money you save when you cut down on hospital visits. In fact, consider how much money you save just by cutting down on Over the Counter drugs that are so common when you have frequent wheezing from a polluted environment; or even irritated skin from the chemical triggered allergies. This is money that becomes available to improve your quality of life in other more pleasant ways.

Food that is clear of artificial preservatives and also additives. You will be pleased to know that the organizations that are charged with the role of certifying organic foods also restrict the use of additives and artificial preservatives in packed foods. This is a way of ensuring that your naturally produced food is not interfered with at the last stages; maintaining the organic status of the food.

By choosing to eat organically, you can avoid a lot of GMO's and pesticides that are a normal part of our food. There are so many pesticides used that it is estimated that the average American consumes 16 pounds of pesticides a year through the food that they eat. Organic food is free of these pesticides. Organic food farmers use tried and true farming methods. They manage and nourish their soil, they don't use pesticides and they avoid GMO foods. Because of these basic farming practices, the food not only avoids the contamination of pesticides but it actually has more nutrients and even tastes better than non-organic food. It may be hard to switch to an organic lifestyle mainly because it is more expensive. Your expense is justified in that you are spending more to help support a more sustainable lifestyle. In addition, you can cut the cost of your food by growing and eating your own food from your own garden.

Organic farmers used tried and true farming practices. These farming practices use nutrient-rich soil. By growing food in nutrient-rich soil, in turn, your food that you are consuming also is rich in nutrients. By eating organically, you not only avoid pesticides but you are eating a healthier product, which in turn will help your body get the vitamins and minerals it needs. By practicing your own organic farming methods, you can benefit from this healthier lifestyle.

Non-Organic foods

GMOs are not organic because really, farmers of GMOs really babysit them; spraying herbicides to protect them against fluctuating weather conditions, and such other chemical-related treatments that ensure a bumper harvest. How about those internal processes that ensure that a GMO tomato is smoother and glossier than a baby's cheek, and a carrot is as straight and smooth as nothing else could be? Are those not scientific processes that distort the organic make-up of the product? For sure, GMOs cannot pass the organic test.

Genetically Modified Organisms (or GMOs) have swept the world of consumption and biotechnology industry in a very controversial manner. The term itself has prompted several countries to ban their production. Many skeptical consumers have likewise challenged state laws in making GMO labeling mandatory in all food products sold on the market.

And not only will you be better advised to keep off GMOs, you will also be asked to be keen if farms in the neighborhood are growing

GMOs. The reason is that a lot of cross-pollination takes place, mostly through the wind, and organic crops in the neighborhood are likely to be thus polluted.

In addition, the effect of strong pesticides is likely to also find its way to neighboring organic farms. So, when you go shopping, even as you read the label that indicates that the food is organic, have a look at its source. If you have more than one option, go for the option whose source is in a neighborhood famous for organic farms. Playing safe in matters of healthy eating is not arrogance; it is only being proactive in a bid to live a longer and healthier life.

In short, organic foods are foods you will not worry about even when you eat them raw; in any case, there is no evil within that you are trying to kill through fire. But with natural foods, we see nobody trying to vouch for them. If we are to eat them, we can only rely on hope. In fact, if you think of ordinary water, which in any case we deem natural, is it of any nutritional value to you? Of course it is not.

Water is good alright, because it helps you sweat out excess salts and do a few more things that make you comfortable, but it will not add any vitamins, proteins, and such other nutrients to your body. So, much as natural foods are not necessarily bad, they do not fall under the realm of foods whose benefits you can evaluate before sale.

Eating organic is not just for the rural folk to whom this kind of eating comes more or less naturally. It is something that has become the in-thing, particularly to those that are enlightened in matters of health. But, granted, organic eating did not begin as the first choice for the rich and famous – no. For many years, moneyed people ate a sophisticated diet that was dominated by processed non-organic foods. Then ailments emerged; and doctors became more and more concerned as they realized that some of the serious ailments emerging are as a result of inorganic diet. And thus came the wisdom of organic eating.

Difference Between Organic and Non-organic Foods?

The first one is that organic food is grown using natural fertilizer. The inorganic one is grown using synthetic fertilizers.

The second difference is that pest control is through natural means such as the use of birds, traps, insects, or natural pesticides. On the other hand, the inorganic ones have pests controlled using synthetic fertilizers.

The third one that you should be conscious of is that animal products like eggs, milk and meat are free from GMOs and hormones. Livestock reared under inorganic conditions are fed hormones to grow faster.

Fighting diseases under organic involves zero-grazing, rotational grazing and so on. Under the non-organic, medications such as antibiotics are used.

Lastly, the livestock under the organic farming are enclosed or confined. On the other hand, the non-organic ones are free to roam.

This has ultimately made organic foods become one of the fastest growing sectors of the American Food Industry today.

Reasons to Say NO to non-organic food

Allergic reaction and adverse immune responses. Mice which were fed with alpha-amylase inhibitor (insecticidal protein) sustained a strong immunity against GM protein. Antibodies were developed, which allowed the hypersensitivity reaction to delay. This means that the insecticidal protein acts as a sensitizer, which made the mice more susceptible to developing allergies as compared to consuming non-allergenic type of food.

Presence of lesions in the stomach. Ulcers and stomach lesions developed in rats that were fed with GM tomatoes for a period of 28 days. More disturbingly, the study found unexplained deaths among 20% of the 40 rats used in the laboratory test. This particular study was commissioned by the company Calgene, the producer of the GMO tomato called Flavr Savr.

Aging of the liver. Another experiment carried out utilized GM soy fed to mice for a period of 2 years. The result showed rapid changes in the hepatocyte metabolism. Moreover, indications of liver aging such as calcium signaling and stress response changes were found. Mice, which were fed with non-GMO soy showed complete normal liver function.

Dense uterine lining. For a period of 15 months, female rats were given genetically engineered soy. At the end of the test period, results show significant thickening in the lining of the uterus. Additionally, the study recorded changes in the ovaries of these mice as compared to those who took non-GMO soy. The lining of the uterus, also referred to as the epithelium, had higher number of cells.

Unstable functioning of the pancreas, testes, and liver. The internal organs of mice fed with GMO soy demonstrated instability, particularly for the pancreas, testes, and liver. After tests were conducted, scientists have found that there was an abnormal formation of nuclei and nucleoli among the liver cells.

Presence of toxins in the liver and kidney. There are now 19 different studies showing the effects of GMO soy and Bt Maize in mammals. Among the most disturbing results is the consistent and heavy presence of toxins in the liver and kidneys. Long-term feeding trials are currently under-way to validate the chronicity of this condition.

Altered gut bacteria formation and blood biochemistry. Using GMO rice for 90 days, rats demonstrated an increased water intake. These GMO rice-fed rats displaced unstable blood biochemistry. Presence of altered bacteria in the gut was observed, which could consequently lead to disturbed digestive system functions and inefficient nutrition absorption.

Enlarged liver. Monsanto GM canola was used in another study involving rats. For a period of four weeks, these rats developed enlarged organs, particularly the liver. Abnormal increase in the liver size is a sign of toxicity.

How to Make Sure you get the right nutrients

One thing that can be difficult for a lot of people during an intermittent fast is to make sure that they get enough nutrition into their diet when they limit their eating window. The more that you limit your window, the harder it can be to come up with enough nutrition to keep the body healthy. The trick here is to really plan out your days and be mindful of the foods that you are eating during your eating window.

To start, you need to find a calculator or another tool that can help you figure out the number of calories that you should consume every day. This will give you a base number that goes off how many calories you burn just by breathing and being alive, and then adds on for your current height and weight and makes changes based on how active you are during the day. Many of these calculators will also make adjustments to help you figure out a safe caloric amount to go with when you want to lose weight.

Once you have this number, it is time to get planning. You should be able to base your macronutrients from this information as well. You will know exactly how many carbs, fats, and proteins you can have based on your caloric allowance and the diet plan that you want to go on.

Now you need to get to meal planning. We will discuss more about meal planning later on, but this is a great tool to use to help you make sure that you are getting enough nutrients into your day. You can decide how many meals and snacks you want to have during the day and then divide up the nutrients from there. Depending on your eating window, you may want to divide this up between two to three meals. Those on the Warrior diet may even reduce this down to just one meal for the day.

One thing to note here is that many people find themselves very hungry when they get done with a fast, whether they do a daily fast or an alternate day fast. It is best to set up your calories in a way that you can eat more during that first meal after a fast. This helps you to deal with the hunger and cravings you may have right away when the fast ends and won't make you fall off your plan if you just have to have some more. Then, with the other meals and snacks of the day, you can cut down on the calories by just a bit and still stay within your caloric allowance.

When picking out your meal plan, you should include a lot of variety in each meal. This ensures that you will keep your body healthy and will get all the nutrients that you need. When you look at your plate, see all the colors of the rainbow there. This is the easiest way to make sure all the nutrients are covered, without having to go through and find out the nutrients in each item of food. If you are at a loss of which meals to make that will provide your body with a lot of nutrients and will fill you up during your limited eating window, then you can invest in some recipe books and look online to find recipes that have lots of nutrients and will give you the best results from your intermittent fast.

When to eat on a fast day?

For a lot of people, fasting all day long and having a good meal in the evening is the best plan for a fast day. If your calorie allowance is around 500 calories on a fasting day, then you can have one meal that's worth 500 calories at the end of the day. You also have the option of having mini-meals throughout the day; as long as you stick to the calorie restriction. If you follow the crescendo method of fasting, then you will fast on two or three days of the week and eat like you usually would on all the other days. On the days that you fast, you can eat after your fasting window ends. It means that you can eat after you complete 12-16 hours of fasting. After you break your fast, you can have a light meal and follow it later with one or two meals. As mentioned, there are different forms of fasting that you can follow so select one that suits your needs. If you like to have a heavy dinner, then you can save up your calories from the rest of the day and indulge yourself at night. A lot of people find it easier to wait until the evening to have a proper meal. If you think you can do without the meal, then please do so! When you fast throughout the day, you might notice that your body is running low on fuel. In such a case, you can have a salty snack like a handful of popcorn!

Best foods to have

• All Legumes and Beans – good carbs can help lower body weight without planned calorie restriction

• Anything high in protein – helpful in keeping your energy levels up in your efforts as a whole, even when you're in a period of fasting

• Anything with the herbs cayenne pepper, psyllium, or dried/crushed dandelion – they'll contribute to weight loss without sacrificing calories or effort

• Avocado – a high-good-calorie fruit that has a lot of healthy fats

• Berries – often high in antioxidants and vitamin C as well as flavonoids for weight loss

• Cruciferous Vegetables – broccoli, cauliflower, Brussels sprout, and more, are incredibly high in fiber, which you'll want to keep constipation at bay with IF

• Eggs – high in protein and great for building muscle during IF periods

• Nuts & Grains – sources of healthy fats and essential fiber

• Potatoes – when prepared in healthy ways, they satiate hunger well and help with weight loss

• Wild-Caught Fish – high in healthy fats while providing protein and vitamin D for your brain

When it comes to liquids:

• Water:

• It's always good for you! It will help keep you hydrated, it will provide relief with headaches or lightheadedness or fatigue, and it clears out your system in the initial detox period.

•   Try adding a squeeze of lemon, some cucumber or strawberry slices, or a couple of sprigs of mint, lavender, or basil to give your water some flavor if you're not enthused with the taste of it, plain.

•   If you need something other than water to drink, you can always seek out:

•   Probiotic drinks like kefir or kombucha

•   You can even look for probiotic foods such as sauerkraut, kimchi, miso, pickles, yogurt, tempeh, and more!

•   Probiotics work amazingly well at healing your gut, especially in times of great transition, as with the start of intermittent fasting.

•   Black coffee

•   Sweeteners and milk aren't productive for your fasting and weight loss goals.

•   Try black coffee whenever possible, in moderation.

•   Heated or chilled vegetable or bone broths

•   Teas of any kind

•   Apple cider vinegar shots

•   Instead, try water or other drinks with ACV mixed in.

Drinks to avoid

• Regular soda

• Diet soda

• Alcohol of any kind

• Anything with artificial sweetener

• Artificial sweetener will shock your insulin levels into imbalance with your blood sugar later on.

Eating frequency

People believe that continuous snacking helps to keep hunger at bay and reduces the chances of excessive hunger. Frequent meals will naturally leave you feeling full, but you don't have to do this. If you want to cut your cravings and keep hunger at bay, then you'll want to make sure that you are filling yourself up with the right kind of food. Your meals should contain high amounts of fiber, protein, and healthy fats instead of carbs. A meal that's rich in carbs will make you feel hungry soon and make you want to eat more food. Consuming carbs can make you crave more carbs. So, a balanced meal is the key to reducing your hunger.

Being in a fed state continuously isn't natural for the human body. During evolution, humans had to endure periods of starvation. If frequent meals were essential for survival, then the human race would have been wiped out a long time ago. Fasting helps to induce cellular repair by kick-starting the process of autophagy. It helps to protect against diseases like Alzheimer's and even certain types of cancers. Fasting is quite beneficial for the system, and it helps to cleanse the system by eliminating the build-up of toxins in the body. Snacking often has certain disadvantages. Frequent meals can quickly increase your calorie intake and lead to a build-up of fatty cells in the liver.

CHAPTER 16:

Can Intermittent Fasting Be Dangerous

Although most people can follow the intermittent fasting diet with minimal side effects and virtually no lasting side effects, some people might find themselves experiencing some. The most likely dangers that you could experience includes:

You Might Struggle to Maintain Blood Sugar Levels

Although the intermittent fasting diet tends to improve blood sugar levels in most people, this is not always true for everyone. Some people who are eating following the intermittent fasting diet may find that their ability to maintain a healthy blood sugar level is compromised.

The reason for why this happens varies. For some people, not eating frequently enough may encourage this to happen. For others, transitioning too quickly or taking on too intense of a fasting cycle too soon, can shock the body which in turn causes a strange fluctuation in blood sugar levels.

You Might Experience Hormonal Imbalances

A certain degree of fasting, especially when you build up to it, can support you in having healthier hormone levels. However, for some people, intermittent fasting may lead to an unhealthy imbalance of hormones. This can result in a whole slew of different hormone-based symptoms, such as headaches, fatigue, and even menstrual problems in women.

Again, the reason for the hormonal imbalance varies. For some people, particularly those who are already at risk of experiencing hormonal imbalances, intermittent fasting can trigger these imbalances to take place. For others, it could go back to what they are consuming during the eating windows. Eating meals that are not rich in nutrients and vitamins can result in you not having enough nutrition to support your hormonal levels.

If you begin experiencing hormonal imbalances when you eat the intermittent fasting diet, it is essential that you stop and consult your doctor right away. Discovering where the shortcomings are and how you can correct them is vital. Having imbalanced hormones for too long can lead to diseases and illnesses that require constant life-long attention.

Headaches

A decrease in your blood sugar level and the release of stress hormones by your brain as a result of going without food are possible causes of headaches during the fasting window. Problems may also be a clear message from your body telling you that you are very low on water and getting dehydrated. This may happen if you are completely engrossed in your daily activities, and you forget to drink the required amount of water your body needs during fasting.

To handle headaches, ensure you stay well hydrated throughout your fasting window. Keep in mind that exceeding the required amount of water per day may also result in adverse effects. Reducing your stress level can also keep headaches away.

Some people find that the transitioning period includes many headaches. These headaches are often a result of you being hungry as your body adjusts to your new eating schedule. Typically, these headaches are dull and should be manageable. If it is not, you may be experiencing excessively low blood sugars. If your headache is too intense, refrain from fasting and eat. It is better to skip your fasting cycle and eat if you are experiencing negative side effects, than it is to attempt to stick it out and experience adverse or potentially dangerous side effects.

If you are experiencing chronic headaches, you may also be experiencing dehydration. Dehydration is common in most people, but it can be especially prevalent in those who are fasting. Typically, eating encourages us to drink, too. This is how we "wash it down." When you are not eating, you may also forget to drink water. Setting reminders to drink water and remember to get at least 3L a day can support you in overcoming headaches that may be caused by dehydration.

Cravings

During your fasting periods, you might find that you have higher levels of desires than usual. This often happens because you are telling yourself that you cannot have any food, so suddenly you start craving many different foods. This is because all you are thinking about is food. As you think about food, you will begin to think about the different types of food that you like and that you want. Then, the cravings start.

Early on, you may also find yourself craving more sweets or carbs because your body is searching for an energy hit through glucose. While you do not want to have excessive levels of sugar during your eating window, as this is bad for blood sugar, you can always have some. The ability to satisfy your cravings is one of the benefits of eating a diet that is not as restrictive as some other foods are.

From a psychological angle, cravings are intensified because of a feeling of being deprived of what you love to eat. For example, telling you to keep away from eating chocolate will somehow make you want to eat chocolate even more because you are unconsciously trying to overcome the feeling of being deprived. Stopping yourself from eating at the usual times you have conditioned your body to received food will naturally make you crave food more at those typical eating times.

To effectively handle your cravings, keep your mind off of food during the fasting window. Ensure that during your eating window, you indulge a bit with what your body craves. This will help to dampen the longing for that thing. Remember that you are not dieting, but fast, so you shouldn't worry unnecessarily over what you eat. Your focus should be on when you eat.

Low Energy

A feeling of lethargy is not uncommon during fasting, especially at the start. This is your body's natural reaction to switching its source of energy from glucose in your meals to fat stored in your body. So, expect to feel a little less energized in your first few weeks of starting with intermittent fasting.

To troubleshoot the feeling of lethargy, try as much as possible to stay away from overly strenuous activities. Keep things low key. Spending more time sleeping or just relaxing is another right way to ensure that your energy reserves are not depleted too quickly. The first few weeks are not the time to test your limits or push yourself.

Foul Mood

You may find yourself being on edge during fasting, even if you are someone who is naturally predisposed to being good-natured. The reason for the feeling of edginess is straightforward. You are hungry, yet you won't eat, and you are struggling to keep your cravings in check, plus, you may already be feeling tired and sluggish. Add all of these to the internal hormone changes due to the sharp decline in your blood sugar levels, and it's no wonder why you may be in such a foul mood. Tempers can easily flare up, and you may be quick to become irritated. This is normal when beginning a fasting lifestyle.

To effectively troubleshoot this, do all you can to keep away from irritable people and situations. If you consider someone annoying, do your best to stay out of their company or else they are more than likely to set you on edge. Find a way to deliberately focus your attention on things that easily trigger a feeling of happiness in you. Consciously seeking ways to be appreciative of the things around you, as well as to being grateful about the simple things of life, will go a long way toward keeping you from being easily irritated.

To handle this cold feeling, you can put on extra warm clothing, stay in friendly places, or drink a hot cup of unsweetened coffee. Taking a hot shower can also reduce the coldness.

Excess Urination

Fasting tends to make you visit the bathroom more frequently than usual. This is an expected side effect since you are drinking more water and other liquids than before. Avoiding water to reduce the number of times you use the bathroom is not a good idea at all, no matter how you look at it. Cutting down water intake while you are fasting will make your body become dehydrated very quickly. If that happens, losing weight will be the least of your problems. Whatever you do, do not avoid drinking water when you are fasting. Doing that is paving the way for a humongous health disaster waiting to happen. You don't want to do that.

The best way to handle excess urination is to stay close to a bathroom or a toilet wherever you find yourself throughout the day. You should urinate when the need arises. There is no other healthy shortcut to it.

People who are intermittently fasting tend to drink a lot of water in between eating windows. That is if they remember to. Often, water is used as a way to fill up your stomach to avoid feeling hungry throughout the day. It can also support you in overcoming heartburn. As a result, water is a popular option for people who are intermittently fasting.

At first, you may even find yourself going as often as twice an hour! There truly is no way around this, as water is essential and you do not want to decrease your intake. This will likely be a symptom that you experience on an ongoing basis, but you should see it as a good sign. This proves that you are well-hydrated and taking good care of your body.

Heartburn, Bloating, and Constipation

Your stomach is responsible for producing stomach acid, which is used to break down food and trigger the digestion process. When you eat frequent meals, unusually large meals, regularly, your body is used to producing high amounts of stomach acid to break down your food. As you transition to a fasting diet, your stomach has to get used to not producing as much stomach acid.

You might also notice an increase in constipation and bloating. People who eat regularly consume high amounts of fiber and proteins that support a healthy digestion process. When you switch to the intermittent fasting cycle, you can still eat a high volume of fiber and protein. However, early on, you might find that you forget to. As you discover the right eating habits that work for you, it may take some time for you to get used to finding ways to work in enough fiber and protein to keep your digestion flowing.

Heartburn may not be a widespread adverse effect, but it does sometimes occur in some individuals. Your stomach produces highly concentrated acids to help break down the foods you consume. But when you are fasting, there is no food in your stomach to be broken down, even though acids have already been produced for that purpose. This may lead to heartburn.

Bloating and constipation usually go hand in hand and can be very discomforting to individuals who suffer from it due to fasting.

Heeding the advice to drink adequate amounts of water usually keeps bloating and constipation in check. Heartburn typically resolves itself quickly, but you can take an antacid tablet or two if it persists. You may also consider eating fewer spicy foods when you break your fast.

You Might Experience Low Energy and Irritability

Until now, your body has been used to having a constant stream of energy pouring in all day long. From the time you wake up until the time you go to bed, it has been receiving some form of power from the foods that you eat. So, when you stop eating regularly, your body grows confused. It has to learn to create its energy rather than rely on the heat being offered to it by the food that you are eating.

Depending on how you are eating, your body may also be growing used to consuming fat as a fuel source rather than carbohydrates. This means that, in addition to losing its primary energy source, it also has to switch how it consumes energy and where it comes from. This can lead to lowered energy for a while. Do things that exert the least amount of energy. If you are someone who regularly exercises and works out, reducing the amount that you work out or switching to a more relaxed workout like yoga can help you during the transition period.

You Might Start Feeling Cold

As you begin to adjust to your intermittent fasting diet, you might find that your fingers and toes get quite cold. This happens because blood flow towards your fat stores is increasing, so blood flow to your extremities reduces slightly. This supports your body in moving fat to your muscles so that it can be burned as a fuel to keep your energy levels up.

Lowered blood sugars from fasting can also lead to cold extremities. More so, it makes them feel more sensitive to the cold. Staying warm with tea, hot showers, and extra layers can help overcome this coldness. If you notice that it is particularly prominent or that it spreads beyond your fingers and toes, you might want to adjust your diet to ensure that you are not experiencing chronic low blood sugars. This will ensure that you continue effectively managing your symptoms without experiencing adverse or dangerous side effects from intermittent fasting.

You Might Find Yourself Overeating

The chances for overeating during the break of the fast are high, especially for beginners. Understandably, you will feel starving after going without food for longer than you are used to. It is this hunger that causes some people to eat hurriedly and surpass their standard meal size and average caloric intake. For others, overeating may be as a result of uncontrollable appetite. Hunger may push some people to prepare too much food for breaking their fast, and if they don't have a grip on their desire, they will continue to eat even when they are satiated. Overeating or binging when you break your fast will make it difficult to reach your goal of optimal health and fitness.

An excellent way to tackle this is by making adequate plans ahead of time and sticking to those plans. Plan the quantity of food to be prepared well ahead of the eating window. Take into consideration the type of food as well as the meal size to be eaten. Although it may not be feasible to continually eat only fatty foods, increasing the frequency as well as the number of healthy fats in your diet will help you to feel satiated quickly.

During the windows where you can eat, you might find yourself eating as much as you possibly can. This is often a natural response to the feelings of hunger that you have experienced during your fasting cycle.

Choosing healthier options and eating mindfully is a good way to overcome overeating habits. This can support you in selecting options that are going to nourish and help your body, as well as prevent overeating. When you eat slowly and mindfully, you can recognize when you are no longer hungry. As a result, you can set down the fork and stop eating. Eating healthier options and eating slowly are the best ways to avoid overeating so that you do not waste your fasting benefits on an excessively unhealthy diet during your eating windows.

Hunger Pangs

People who start intermittent fasting may initially feel quite hungry. This is especially common if you are the type of person who tends to eat regular meals daily.

If you start feeling hungry, you can choose to wait it out if you have an eating window right around the corner. However, if there is a more extended waiting period or you are feeling excessively hungry, you should eat. Feeling hungry to the point that it becomes uncomfortable or distracting is not helpful and will not support you in successfully taking on the intermittent fasting diet. This is a pronounced side effect of going without food for longer than you are accustomed to.

For many people, their bodies have been conditioned to eat at certain regular intervals. So, at those intervals, their hunger hormones kick into action and stimulate a feeling of hunger. They either respond by eating a full meal or grabbing a quick snack. It is almost impossible not to feel very hungry when you attempt to break this pattern. Introducing fasting into your lifestyle is going to make you hungry. There are no two ways about it, and I'm not going to lie to you. The intensity of hunger is even higher when you are just starting. Hunger tests your resolve and mental toughness, especially in your first few days. This is the point where many will give up and walk away from their dreams and aspirations. But if you stay true to your resolve, hunger has a way of waning over time.

To reduce the hunger pangs, keep yourself occupied in some way throughout your fasting window. Keeping yourself busy, in addition to drinking water whenever you feel bouts of hunger, will help to keep your mind off food as well as suppress the appetite. Another way to troubleshoot hunger is to make sure you eat enough healthy fats, proteins, and fiber the day before you begin fasting.

The method of fasting that you opt for is entirely up to you. Hunger pangs are quite familiar during the initial week of fasting; don't get scared. Your body isn't used to starvation, and it will take a while to condition yourself to the diet. A hunger pang doesn't always indicate hunger. Confusing isn't it? At times, you will feel hungry when you are stressed or even bored. It is essential that you realize the difference between actual hunger and a natural craving. Ignore these pangs and get on with your day. Intermittent fasting doesn't mean that you should starve yourself, but at the same time, you shouldn't indulge in mindless eating either.

CHAPTER 17:

How To Stay Motivated When Practicing Intermittent Fasting

The first couple of weeks of intermittent fasting cannot only be hard as heck, but it can also sometimes be a little disappointing if you don't see any tangible results from your hard work. This can make it almost impossible for some women to stay motivated, especially if they see the scale go up in those first uncomfortable weeks.

Find a fasting buddy

It is easier to keep going when you know there is someone else fasting with you. It can be your husband, best friend, or family member. Sit down with them and walk them through the basics of the intermittent fasting technique you have chosen. Use each other as support on those days when one of you doesn't feel like fasting or exercising. It will be more fun when you have someone who you can plan meals with, shop for food with, train with and learn with.

Set achievable goals

It is best to start with short-term goals that you know you can achieve. Once you attain that goal, reward yourself, but don't do it with junk food. This will help boost your momentum and motivation.

Keep a progress journal

This is a great way to look at the positive changes you have been experiencing ever since you started your fast. Get a diary and start writing how you feel and all the progress you are making. It is essential to take time to look at how your body and life is transforming. Look at how your clothes fit, the energy you now have to play with your kids, and the way your sleep has improved. Track your positive progress and whip out that journal whenever you feel yourself losing motivation.

Don't beat yourself up

Yes, there are days when you will fail and succumb to temptation. Things will get rough, and you will grab a cookie and start munching away. Be compassionate with yourself. Don't start talking negatively about yourself just because you didn't do things right.

Pray and meditate

When you start to feel discouraged, take some time to feed and strengthen your soul and spirit. Pray, read scriptures, and meditate. This will help you love yourself despite the challenges you face in life.

Focus On the Good

Throughout the first few weeks, I'm betting that you've found yourself with more energy, especially following the feeding phase, had heightened alertness, euphoria, and even creativity. That felt great, didn't it? You've likely also had more time on your hands recently, particularly so if you are skipping a meal that you usually would spend a bit of time preparing. What does that extra time allow you to do? While you may not notice significant observable weight loss within those first few days and weeks of intermittent fasting, there is always a good point you can focus on. Think about the extra time that you're getting with your family or loved ones, all the extra stuff you're getting done, and how it's helping you at work to stay motivated when you're not seeing those quick results that you were hoping for. Usually, after week three or four is when you start to see the beginning of fat loss, and its generally pretty steady from there.

Go slow

These changes take a while, and they do not happen overnight. If you want to lose weight and make sure that it stays at bay, then you'll need to lose weight slowly. You can starve yourself and shed a few pounds, but it will not do you any good. The more gradual and steady your weight loss, the easier it is to maintain. Intermittent fasting is a great dieting option, and it is sustainable. Make sure you go slowly. There is no hurry, and you don't need to jump right in.

Be Your Coach

You are the best person to motivate yourself. You can program your mind to think precisely what you want it to think. You need to drive yourself by positively reinforcing your efforts and reminding yourself of your motivational reasons. Each day, you can program your mind and body to become an incredible fat-burning machine. When you use these self-motivational methods, your brain will believe everything you tell yourself.

Be Willing to Forgive Yourself

Don't forget, Intermittent Fasting is not a walk in the park. You may realize it's not as easy as people make it out to be. Perhaps you choose to attend a birthday party, and in the process, you ate delicious food instead of sticking to your fasting schedule. That's fine. Just remember, do not beat yourself up about it because this is normal and you're only human. Instead of punishing yourself, realize the mistake, and immediately get back on track and move forward.

Setbacks are common

Temptation can strike, and there will be times when you might give in to your lures. After all, you are only human. It is okay to face a setback, but don't think of it as a failure. The attitude with which you deal with a delay can set the course for the rest of your diet.

Be patient

One of the significant obstacles to a diet is the weight loss plateau. You might eat right and exercise correctly, but the numbers on the scales don't seem to change. The scale appears to be stuck for some reason. Well, this is known as the weight-loss plateau, and it is something that every dieter faces. Merely turn around and congratulate yourself for your success so far. It is a part of the process of weight loss.

Reward yourself

Dieting does take some effort, and it might not seem fun at times. So don't forget to treat yourself when you achieve a goal. A goal could be big or small. When you reach your goal, you should treat yourself. The reward doesn't have to be an extravagant one. Perhaps you can buy yourself a bottle of nail polish that you wanted! The rewards you set for yourself should never be food-related. Don't reward yourself with a pint of ice cream for losing 5 pounds in ten days. It doesn't make any sense and renders the diet redundant. When you celebrate your success, it will make you feel better about yourself and your food. Also, it will provide you with the necessary motivation to keep going even when you want to give up.

CHAPTER 18:

Starter Meal Plan

When you choose to start eating on an intermittent fasting cycle, it is always important to make sure that you make the transition at a pace that is manageable by your body. Attempting to transition too quickly can result in negative side effects that can be extremely challenging to deal with, including the side effects mentioned in Chapter 4.

Before you begin the intermittent fasting diet, take some time to learn what your natural eating pattern is. Spending just a few days discovering how you naturally eat can support you in understanding what you need to transition successfully. Even if you already have a fairly good idea of what your natural eating pattern is, you should still spend a few days purposefully documenting it.

As you document your natural eating pattern, take the time to look at both when you typically eat and what you typically eat. Also note down what you are craving, especially if what you are craving is different from what you actually ate. This will give you important information as to what your natural eating cycles are so that you can transition in a way that presents minimal shock to your body.

When you begin eating the intermittent fasting diet, start slowly and pay attention to your symptoms. Do not attempt to set a time frame as to when you will move on to the next phase as this might result in you pushing yourself too quickly. Alternatively, you might find yourself waiting too long and wasting time.

When you know what you need and what you can handle, picking the right diet that is going to serve your health goals and keep you feeling great is much easier.

Avoid eating more than you need to, but do not hesitate to eat what you need. The idea of intermittent fasting is for you to fast, not starve. This means that you are simply not eating, not that you are not feeling a complete sense of starvation. Knowing how to keep yourself in a fast without feeling like you are truly starving takes time and practice, so be patient with yourself and keep trying. You will get the hang of it as your body acclimates more.

Whenever an eating window arrives, seek to eat as healthy as possible. While there are no exact requirements on what you should eat, choosing healthier food choices is going to support your transition phase in a big way. Many people who experience intense episodes of headaches or other symptoms are experiencing them because they are not nourishing their body properly in between fasts.

Eating a healthy diet in between will ensure that your body is being nourished with all of the vitamins and minerals that it needs to operate healthfully. This will support healthy bodily functions, thus promoting the benefits of fasting rather than working against it. While this does not mean that you should completely avoid dessert or ditch any and all unhealthy snacks, it does mean that you should opt for healthier options whenever possible.

When you choose healthier options, this will not only support you in feeling better during your fasting cycles but it will also support you in achieving your goals. Your healthier options will help you in experiencing greater energy levels, improved weight loss, increased muscle gain, and better overall health. As a result, your diet and your eating cycles will both work together to help you achieve your goals faster and with greater sustainability.

It is important that you refrain from eating excessive levels of sugar when you are intermittently fasting. This includes avoiding excessive levels of processed and artificial sugars in addition to avoiding excessive levels of natural sugars. One of the wonderful benefits of intermittent fasting is that you can level out your blood sugar levels. However, you want to maintain these balanced out levels.

When you are intermittently fasting, a good idea is to avoid high carb intake altogether. Eating a low-carb or ketogenic diet can support you in getting all of the nutrition that you need without consuming carbohydrates as a filler. This will not only support you in avoiding the unwanted side effects but will also ensure that you are gaining the maximum value of your diet. Lowering your carbohydrates will actually increase the level of ketones in your body, making it even easier for you to experience increased energy, weight loss, and muscle gain.

Increasing your intake of healthy fats throughout your eating windows can support your body in having plenty of fats to produce energy from. It is important that you choose healthy fats for this, as this will keep your fuel clean and effective. Filling up on unhealthy fats can be dangerous as it can actually have a negative impact on heart and blood health. Fats like the ones you get from avocado oil and coconut oil, nuts and seeds, fish, and cheeses can support you in maintaining your energy and staying healthy while eating the intermittent fasting diet. I have included a list of healthy fats below to give you an idea of what to look for and where to start.

Sugary and starchy foods should be avoided in any diet. They can reduce metabolic efficiency and cause blood sugar spikes. When you are intermittently fasting, avoiding these types of foods can help you maintain your overall health. It can also support you in reducing negative side effects during your fasting cycles.

3 day-meal plan for a Fat man

As with any diet, intermittent fasting requires commitment and consistency. The benefits of fasting will appear relatively quickly. You'll notice increased energy and focus, better regulation of your diet and schedule. Without any restrictions on the types of foods you can enjoy, intermittent fasting is an ideal option for people who are already happy with their diet yet want to achieve results sooner. Getting the most out of your diet can include choosing healthy, nutritious foods and recipes that are easy to make and delicious. To start fresh with some new meal ideas in between your fasting schedule, the following Meals are examples of healthy, recommended options.

Burning fat, eating well and following intermittent fasting as well as other diets are only part of the solution. One of the biggest obstacles to overcome is loving your own body, regardless of your age, shape or health. In becoming more comfortable in your own skin, confidence grows, along with the success of any diet plan, routine or fitness level, you'll find a major improvement in your life. This will inspire others to embark on the same or similar journeys to achieve success through intermittent fasting.

Below you'll see a sample 3-day meal plan for a very fat man who is yearning to lose weight.

Day1

1. Oatmeal 120g, 1 banana or another fruit.

3. 150g of brown rice (pasta, buckwheat) with 100g of turkey breast with vegetables.

4. 200g of Cottage cheese and 10-15g of nuts (walnuts, peanuts, almonds)

Total: about 1300kcal

Day2

1. 2 whole eggs 2slices of whole-grain bread (40g) with 8olives.

2. 200g of low-fat cottage cheese 30g of blueberries (other berries).

3. 200g of chicken breast with vegetables (stewed zucchini, rhubarb,

and spinach) and a spoon of olive oil..

4. 200g of Greek yogurt and 20g of nuts.

Total: about 1500kcal

Day3

1. 2 eggs, 2 pieces of bread (30g) and half of the avocado.

2. Walnuts 30g

3. 150g of buckwheat and vegetables (tomatoes, cucumber, iceberg, salad)

4. 200g of natural yogurt and 15-20g of nuts (walnuts, peanuts, almonds)

Total: about 1500kca

3-day meal plan for an Average weight woman

Ideally, for a woman to benefit from Intermittent fasting, they should incorporate the following into their choice of meals to break the fast: Carbohydrates – from fruits, vegetables and grains.

It is advisable to make healthy choices within the week as you continue to do Intermittent fasting. If you decide to keep Intermittent fasting as part of your lifestyle or routine, you'll be inclined to prepare or buy healthy meals instead of processed food.

Below you'll see a sample 3-day meal plan for an average weight woman. It consists of healthy choices that are flavorful and appeal to the palate. Feel free to mix and match your choices. Just don't forget to make vegetables and fruit a daily part of your meal.

Day 1

1. 120g Of oatmeal and 1 tablespoon of honey.

2. 120 g Of buckwheat with vegetables (iceberg, cucumbers, carrots)) (one spoon of flaxseed oil on top of that)

3. 2 avocado sandwiches with whole-grain bread and tomato slice on top (use half or regular avocado) (this meal is my favorite)

Total: about 1500kcal

Day 2

1. 400g of pineapple (mango, kiwi)

2. 200g of salmon with vegetables (beetroot, broccoli, carrots, cabbage) (a spoon of olive oil on top)

3. Salad with one avocado and 30g of olives (different kinds of greens included, pick what you want)

Total: about 1400kcal

Day 3

1. 400g of fruit mix (1 banana, apple, ½ of pear)

2. 3 boiled eggs with vegetables(carrots, broccoli, radishes...)

3. 200gof salmon(300g of tuna) with green vegetables and 30 g of olives.

Total: about 1400kcal.

CONCLUSION

Thank you for making it to the end of this book. I hope that you have learned some of the benefits of IF and have a better understanding of intermittent fasting, in some form or another.

You should now understand how intermittent fasting can be beneficial to your health goals.

Whatever the reason you have chosen to explore intermittent fasting, hopefully, you have found the answers you were looking for and a way to reach your goals, whether they are for weight loss and management or to improve your overall health. Keep working on improving yourself, stay informed, and enjoy your new healthy life!

Do not forget that this is a strengthening exercise for your mind and body. Celebrate your wins along the way and do not be discouraged by what you may think of as setbacks. When you dive into intermittent fasting, you should be doing so with the mindset of making a long-term commitment to yourself and your health. This means that the little steps you take forward, in the beginning, will be what leads you to the big success in your future.

The beauty of intermittent fasting is that it is more of a lifestyle as opposed to the normal diet. Intermittent fasting is much less restrictive as it is focusing on when you eat more than what you eat. You can experiment with what fasting protocol best fits you and your lifestyle. Once you have adjusted to a schedule that works for you, there is nothing left but to enjoy feeling good and having the freedom to do and eat what you like.

Intermittent fasting is more of a change in your lifestyle rather than just a diet. If you want sustainable weight loss and want to lose fat along with it, then you should stick to this diet. You can see positive changes in your body within a month of following this diet.

Good luck.

Made in the USA
Monee, IL
03 February 2020

21238854R00085